BOOTS AND FORCEPS

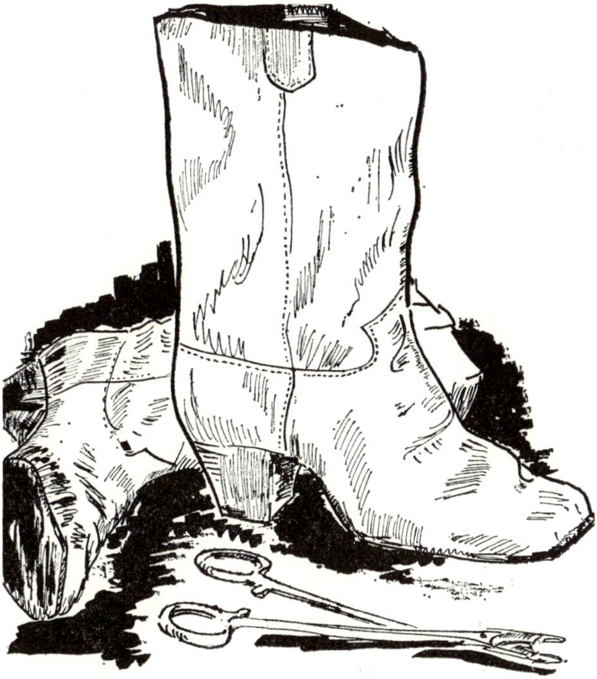

BOOTS AND FORCEPS

WILLET J. PRICE, D.V.M

as told to HAZEL HECKMAN

Drawings by HELEN HIATT

THE IOWA STATE UNIVERSITY PRESS, AMES

1973

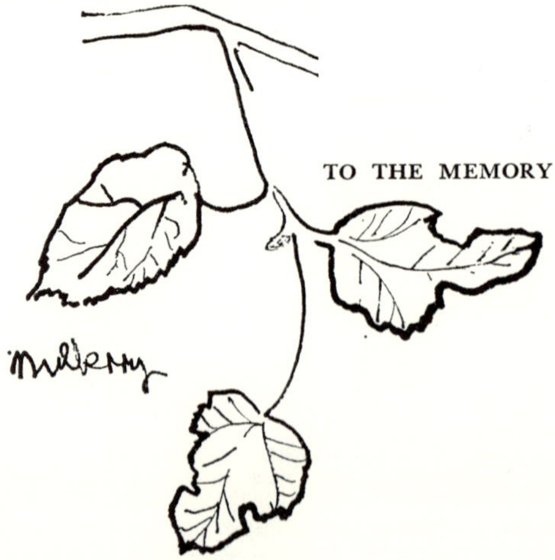

TO THE MEMORY OF OUR MOTHER AND FATHER

WILLET J. PRICE was graduated from Kansas State University with the D.V.M. degree in 1931. He was a practicing veterinarian at Woodward, Oklahoma, 1931–1936, and at Wisner, Nebraska, 1936–1960, except for a time in the Army Veterinary Corps, 1943–1945, when he was stationed at several bases in the Midwest. Because he yearned for the wildness of open range country again he chose to enter government work and was with the USDA Animal Health Division at McGill, Nevada, 1960–1966. In December of 1965 he received a Certificate of Merit for superior performance as USDA district veterinarian in Nevada in work toward the eradication of brucellosis. Facing retirement reluctantly, Dr. Price worked part-time in the profession he loved and in places appealing to him until his full retirement in 1971. He died suddenly on April 10, 1972.

HAZEL HECKMAN, sister of Dr. Price, is a native of Kansas but has lived on Anderson Island, Washington, since 1966. She is author of *Island in the Sound* (1967) and *Island Year* (1972); a short story in *Best Humor Annual;* and fiction and nonfiction in *Harper's, Saturday Evening Post, Farm Journal,* and other magazines. She won the Pacific Northwest Bookseller's Award for nonfiction in 1967 and the Governor's Festival of the Arts Award in 1968.

Composed and Printed by The Iowa State University Press, Ames, Iowa

Library of Congress Cataloging in Publication Data

Price, Willet J 1902–1972.

Boots and forceps.
1. Veterinarians—Correspondence, reminiscences, etc. I. Heckman, Hazel. II. Title.
SF613.P7A3 636.089'092'4 [B] 77-39465
ISBN 0-8138-0265-2

CONTENTS

PREFACE

As I LOOK BACK over four decades of living and working with farm animals as a doctor of veterinary medicine, I marvel at the changes that have come about in rural living during my lifetime. The great lemming migration to the cities and the gradual merging of crop and pasture land into larger and larger acreages in the hands of impersonal and scientific Polk Street farmers and/or housing developers fill me with wonder and misgivings.

As was my boyhood, my working years were spent among farm families whose balanced enterprises made up a nucleus and a way of life. To be sure, a few boys pulled off to follow white- or blue-collar jobs or to enter professions and some farm girls married urban husbands. But during the years prior to World War I and between the two wars, the majority of farm-bred youngsters made use of skills learned at home. Almost invariably a son of the owner remained to farm the home place, which might already have been in the family for more than one generation, and reared his own children there. At the risk of being dismissed as "nostalgic," I will say that it seems to me this made for a pretty good life. Kids on a farm may have had to forego certain cultural and social advantages; but they learned to work gainfully and, I think, happily, and most of them accepted responsibility as a matter of course.

In times of drouth and depression (especially during these times) we saw less real poverty and deprivation on even the hardest-hit farms than we saw among unemployed in the cities. In this book I have depicted rural life as I knew it as a participant and, later, as a practicing large animal veterinarian. As a lover of horses, I am glad to have lived before technology replaced the horse as a member of the family work force. As both laborer and replenisher of the earth, he paid his honest way.

For the fact that much of the following is personal history, I ask the reader's indulgence. In such anecdotes, I have made general use of the pronoun "we" instead of the more personal "I" in order to include my wife Hazel, who worked as hard as I, both during our years of private practice and our association with the Bureau of Animal Industry in government work.

The pursuit of veterinary medicine has changed materially over the past three or four decades. Stock raising has gone gradually from small individual farms into the hands of large and specialized corporations that sometimes employ a single veterinarian retainer for their herds. Because of this and other reasons, many young graduates have turned to small animal work. I certainly do not blame them.

The only well-to-do veterinarians I have known accumulated their estates largely by grooming, treating, and bathing dogs and cats. (While I am on the subject of grooming and bathing: I stubbornly maintain that to ask a doctor of veterinary medicine to wash and clip your poodle is as absurd as to expect your medical doctor to give you a hair cut.) The country is filled with small animal hospitals, most of them well equipped and scrupulously clean. Many of them are elegant. I have no quarrel with these nor with the doctors who administer them. They render a service to the thousands of animal lovers who cherish their pets. I know very little about this kind of business.

I have tried here, rather, to tell the story of the practicing veterinarian as I knew him, a man subject to call day or night, over any kind of roads and in any kind of weather. The practice of veterinary medicine is not without risk and danger of infection or injury. I have known more than one animal doctor to be crippled for life in the performance of his duty. As is a physician, he may be called upon at odd hours and for foolish reasons, sometimes with the hope that he may be able to rectify the treatment of some untrained amateur or the failure of some home remedy. His clientele is among both the poor and the prosperous. If he is conscientious, he does as much charity work as does his counterpart in human medicine.

Surgery or treatment is often carried out under a deplorable lack of sanitation and with the most uncooperative of patients. True, the loss of an animal is a far less momentous matter than is the loss of a human. But the veterinarian works as hard to cure, or to alleviate suffering as the human doctor. And if he is a lover of animals, as are most veterinarians, he will take his failures seriously. I only hope in these pages to acquaint my readers with some of the problems encountered by the general practitioner, especially of my time, and to document some of the changes that have taken place during forty years of practice.

This book is not to be taken as any kind of scientific study and makes no claims as such. From the standpoint of my own experience, the material related here is completely true.

WILLET J. PRICE, D.V.M.

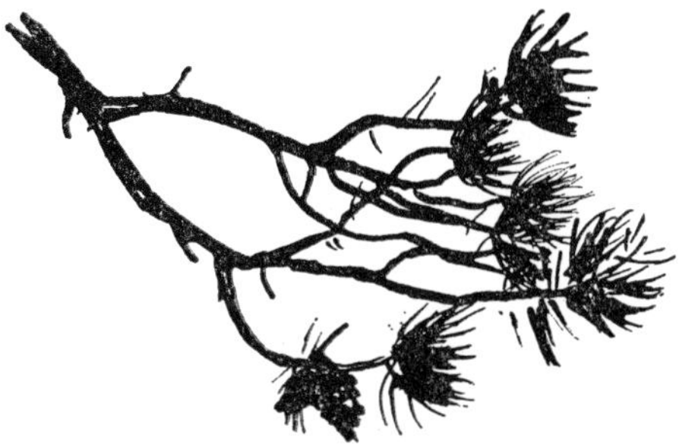

BOOTS AND FORCEPS

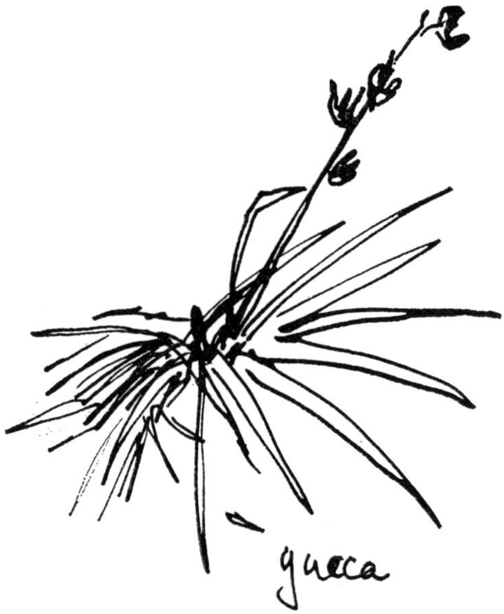

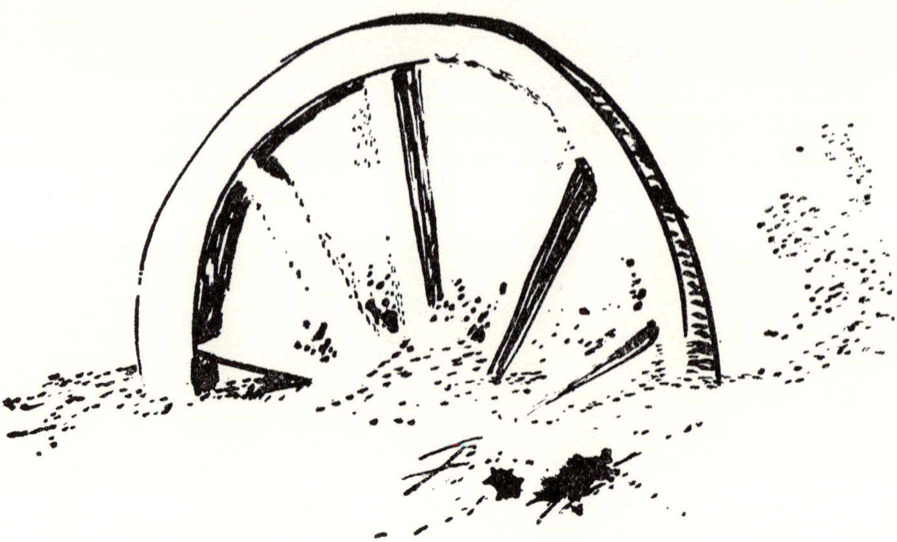

OKLAHOMA

IN A LOCAL NEWSPAPER the other day I came across a photograph that transported me squarely back to a hot August morning in Oklahoma and brought a recollection of the most furious and frightening footrace I have ever been witness to.

The caption on the story read DROUGHT BRINGS MEMORIES OF THE DUSTBOWL. The photograph, dredged out of some Associated Press morgue I reckon, depicted a scene painfully familiar during the time that came to be known among the tormented people of the southwestern part of the United States as "the dirty Thirties." A cluster of farm buildings tied together by a length of rail fence and the four upthrust wheels of a wagon running gear lay more than half buried under mounds and drifts of dust. The cut line read: *Dustbowl Grave of the 1930's.*

As a temporary government employee under orders from the Bureau of Animal Industry, I was engaged in the grisly business of appraising, buying, and slaughtering drouth-stricken and starving cattle around the state. Because the day gave sinister promise of being another scorcher, with limited visibility from the moving pall of dust, I had gone to my assignment early, accompanied by the young Indian whose job it was to finish off the pathetic animals with a knife in order to assure a quick death and to bleed out any meat that was in any way fit for use.

During the bitter days of killing that had gone before, I had grown somewhat accustomed to a small audience of onlookers, generally male. I was hardly prepared for the sight of approximately two hundred men, women, and children armed with kitchen knives we found waiting at the small enclosure on the outskirts of the all-black town where the morning's work was to take place. As the car came to a stop a scared-looking white woman detached herself from a group of women and came toward us.

"I'm from the welfare office," she said uncertainly. "My supervisor sent me out to see that there was a fair division of the meat."

"Well, it looks to me like you've got one hell of a job," I told her. I had long since come to the grim conclusion that my own job fell into the same bracket.

We got through the preliminaries without any disagreement. In this case the appraisal and the payments allotted were simple enough. The animals, under various ownership, came to only about sixty head and we had been instructed to "kill clean." That day we had no live quota. Nor did any of these animals look fit for human consumption. Following the business dealings, I had given the usual orders to "stand clear." But as I raised my gun I was uneasily aware of an air of tense, controlled waiting among the silent blacks.

At the first shot the crowd stampeded. No other word would serve to describe the massed surge forward. As the hopelessly emaciated cow went down, her throat cut expertly by my helper, the dilapidated board fence quivered and the knifewielders were off. I tried to make myself heard. I pled with them to stand back, to wait until the miserable job was finished. But there was no stopping them. My helper beat a hasty retreat to safety.

The flesh disappeared off those old bones as swiftly and as cleanly as though the cow had been attacked by piranhas. Within moments, it seemed, she was reduced to a jumble of hide, hooves, horns, and viscera. Having completed their butchering, those who had been fast enough and fortunate enough to come away with meat streamed past me with their blue, unappetizing-looking burdens. Even the tail was borne away by a thin old man who held it aloft in triumph. The others fell back, but only, I reckoned correctly, to await the demise of the next victim.

I looked about for the white woman who had come to referee the division of the spoils but she was nowhere to be seen. Nor did I see her again. I still do not know how we got through the day without mishap.

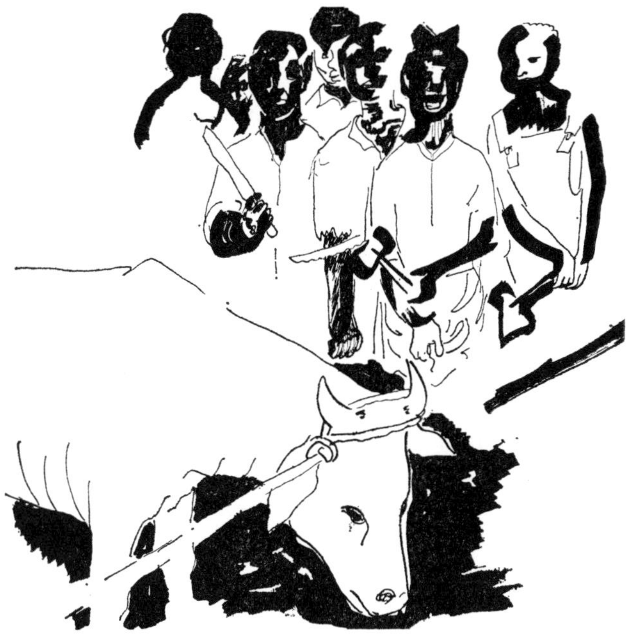

In retrospect, those times and tasks take on the guise of a remembered nightmare. There would be a kind of parallel I suppose in serving as a hangman or in manning an electric chair. Night after night I heard the sound of the gun in my sleep. I had been trained to *save* the lives of animals if possible, not to terminate them on a mass basis. Had I not seen the mercy, the necessity of the program, I could not have carried out the assignment. On one day I killed a total of two hundred and sixty-two animals, a heartbreaking day's work.

My wife, Hazel, and I had chosen Woodward, Oklahoma, as a place to begin practice for a variety of reasons. The population of the town at the time of my graduation from Kansas State Agricultural College in 1931 came to some 5,000 to 6,000 persons. No graduate veterinarian was listed within fifty to one hundred miles in any direction. In the spring of that year a letter had come into the department at school from the widow of a "Doctor Miller" who had been practicing veterinary medicine in the area around Woodward for a number of years. The estate was about to be settled and she wanted to sell the business.

Dr. Miller was not a graduate veterinarian but he had earned the respect and confidence of the farmers and stockmen thereabouts and he was an observing and conscientious practitioner of his chosen vocation. The state of Oklahoma still issued non-graduate licenses on proof of certain qualifications. So far as I know there were no "diploma mills" for veterinarians such as turned out purveyors of human medicine in considerable numbers around the turn of the century. But there were men (and *good* men) who made use of methods and diagnoses learned from their fathers or from earlier practitioners. Men such as Miller supplied the foundation upon which the rest of us were privileged to build.

Other opportunities had come up, including a vacancy at Auburn, Nebraska, in hog country. But, having grown up on a farm in southeast Kansas, I felt more at home in the Southwest. I also preferred working with cattle, and liked the general open-handed friendliness of ranch people. I still do.

Last but not least, Woodward was among the first towns to apply the United States Public Health Service ordinance, was in search of a milk inspector, and was willing to pay thirty dollars a month for the job. A family of three could just about eat on a dollar a day, then.

We paid one hundred and fifty dollars for Dr. Miller's practice, a few instruments, and a small stock of drugs, including some blackleg vaccine. He had devised some kind of healing oil formula for barbed wire cuts, but Mrs. Miller declined to relinquish this. I had passed the Kansas state board examination. I was obliged to pass the Oklahoma board. On July 31, 1931, we set out for Woodward in our second-hand model-T Ford. We would have gone a few weeks earlier had not our four-year-old daughter Marylin, our only child then, come down with measles.

We opened an office in a hardware store, took rooms in the hardware dealer's house, ran an announcement in the local paper, and we were in business.

Woodward does not lie within the strip of counties known as the Oklahoma Panhandle, but it is generally thought of as a Panhandle town. Located in Woodward County, the town lies on the south bank of the North Canadian River, one county removed from Kansas, one county east of the Texas Panhandle. This is sagebrush country, the terrain slightly rolling. You could go twenty-five miles in any direction and find better soil. But the climate is mostly pleasant, with cool nights because of the altitude, and a good deal of wind. Cottonwood and tamarisk and willow trees follow the streams. There is also much mesquite.

I have never forgotten a remark made to me by a client near

one of these shallow streams that dry away to a trickle or nothing at all during a dry summer. He had called me to look at a sick horse. As we sat waiting for the horse to improve, or to die, the anything-but-affluent farmer fell to talking about having made the run in with hundreds of other would-be homesteaders at the opening of the outlet strip.

"My brother and I made the run together," he said. "That is, we *started* the run together. When we got just here and I saw the trees along the stream I reckoned here was wood for free whatever else the country lacked, and so I stopped and set out stakes. Brother kept on a goin'."

I asked how the brother had made out.

The farmer's weathered face crumpled into a wry grin. "He owns three sections down yonder. And I've still got my *wood.*"

There was one thing to be said for having gone through college on a marginal financial basis; the depressed times didn't look much worse than we were accustomed to. Wheat was selling for twenty-five cents a bushel and the prices to be had for other farm products were commensurately low. People are inclined to remember 1929 as a depression year. Actually, 1929 was only the year the stock market broke. The depression hung on for ten years more, and the Panhandle country was further depressed by an extended period of unprecedented drouth.

The area around Woodward was known among ranchers as "cow and calf country." Calves were mostly sold at weaning time, to be shipped to feed yards in the Corn Belt. The only "steer" man we knew was Phil Ferguson, who was to become a United States representative from the district. The Ferguson family owned a good-sized ranch in the Panhandle and another in the Flint Hills of south central Kansas. Steer calves were bought in Texas, run on the range until they attained a weight of around eight hundred pounds, then taken to Kansas to finish off for market. The Oklahoma range consisted largely of buffalo grass.

One of the first friends we made at Woodward was a dairyman named Jack Farrier who helped us to get acquainted with other dairymen and farmers. We tested milk and tested dairy herds for tuberculosis. When a local medical doctor died, we took over his place, a combination office and living quarters, where we tested milk, mixed medicines, sterilized instruments, and treated (and sometimes housed) small animals brought in for diagnosis. This combination had its drawbacks, but Hazel never complained. She knew as much about the testing as I did, kept the books, answered the telephone, met clients, and cared for animals. I couldn't very well have managed without her help.

Considerable rivalry existed among the dairymen concerning the milk tests, a good thing, of course, for the consumer. One producer in particular dropped in often to spy on his competitors' products. Most of the milk was consistently good, but a single incident such as the switch of a tail or a moment of carelessness in utensil cleaning can throw a test a grade off.

Such an accident happened to the snooping dairyman once on a day he chose for dropping in. That day his own sample, generally of the highest grade, was black with sediment. He took one horrified look, bowed his head in shame, and walked out, his hands clasped sadly behind him, as a dog might carry its tail between its legs.

When a drop in buying power resulted in a surplus of milk, dairymen thereabouts sold their product at two quarts for nine cents. I don't think there was any thought of dumping in order to keep the price up as happened elsewhere. Hundreds of gallons of milk were turned over to the welfare agencies, gratis, by men who needed the income for their own livelihood.

Most of the dairies were small family enterprises, with milk drawn by hand and cared for by the womenfolk. As veterinarian as well as inspector, I was once called upon to try to remedy a peculiar condition we called "stringy milk," which occurred after milk had stood overnight in the crocks. "Ropy milk," on the other hand, an indication of bovine mastitis, shows up at the time of milking. Dairymen began to call us to say that something was wrong with the cows.

After the cows checked out healthy, we asked diplomatically whether we might be allowed to examine the kitchen utensils, explaining that even a clean-appearing utensil might cause trouble. You couldn't buy chlorine products at a grocery store then; but we had developed a product of our own. After we had explained its use to the dairy wives as gently as possible, the problem cleared up. We never learned, really, what strange organism lurked in the containers, strainers, buckets, or crocks.

Obliged to make do on a very small budget, we had devised a somewhat ingenious if crude device for injections of a drug to control the occasional bout of mastitis we encountered. This consisted of a syringe attached to a square Ballantine whiskey bottle, of the right size and easy to hold onto. When the bottle fell and broke one day, Hazel visited the liquor store, brought home a bottle of fresh Ballantine, emptied the contents into a quart jar, attached the syringe to the empty, and we were in business again.

In those days, when "jaky" was a threat, any glass fruit jar filled with an amber or clear beverage was suspect. When a colleague dropped in for a visit one day, Hazel produced the quart jar and asked, "Would you like a drink, Doctor?"

He eyed the jar in her hand. "Well, no thanks," he said. "If you don't mind. It's just a matter of policy you understand. I'm sure *yours* is all right. But I find it the better part of wisdom never to *touch* home brew these days."

About the time we thought we had scraped the bottom of the barrel something always seemed to turn up. One day Hazel told me we had a total of nineteen dollars in the bank and that we owed fifteen dollars rent. I worried all night. The next morning the phone rang. The superintendent of the state mental hospital at Supply was calling to say the institution's hogs were falling sick and that some of them were dying. I told him I would be right down.

The ailment wasn't difficult to diagnose. The hogs were dying of cholera. Hoping to save a few, I set to work to vaccinate the well-looking animals and instructed the superintendent to get them into separate quarters. He called in some of the patients to help. One of these, a man in his sixties, beat any high jumper I have ever seen. He would leap over the fence like a deer, not bothering to use the gate.

During subsequent calls to the hospital I came to know this athletic fellow and some of the other patients quite well. They were issued rations of chewing tobacco of a very poor grade, and would cut off bits to share with me. It was pretty awful stuff, but I always accepted these gestures of friendship, for I knew these gifts represented a sacrifice and that they would be offended by a refusal.

Once, called to the hospital to doctor a horse's foot, I asked for a gunny sack to protect the bandage. Dispatched to the barn to bring a sack, the athletic patient was gone for such a long time that I mentioned the matter to the superintendent. "I reckon we better go up there," the superintendent told me. "He's probably forgotten what we sent him for and is up there chinning himself on a cross beam."

Sure enough, we found the errand boy happily chinning and counting, his assignment completely forgotten.

One job I accepted as a public service was that of teaching bacteriology, blood chemistry, and immunology to the student nurses in training at the local hospital. I don't know how much the girls got out of the course, but I found it a lot of fun. Out in all kinds of weather, I had bought myself a pair of pull-on boots that fit pretty tight. When I was obliged to go directly to class one day without stopping at home to change, I wore the boots to a lecture. Seeing that two girls in the front row appeared to be paying special attention, and flattered by their absorption, I expounded at length on the subject matter at hand. When at the end of the lecture one of the pair raised a hand, I asked whether there were questions.

"Not about the lesson, Doctor," she said. "We were just wondering how you get into those boots."

When the time came for the final examination, which I knew the girls were dreading, Hazel and I stuffed one hundred questions into capsules and I asked each girl to draw out ten. They were mostly fine, serious-minded girls who did well on examinations and I'll warrant they made good nurses.

Despite the unpretentious facade of our diggings, we were occasionally mistaken for a medical clinic. One evening when I was at work in the back the doorbell rang. A poorly dressed and obviously nervous young girl asked Hazel whether the doctor were in.

"I'm Doctor Price," I told her.

Her eyes dropped to my cherished but not so very clean boots. "You don't *look* like a doctor," she said suspiciously.

"Not a medical doctor," I said. "A veterinarian." She left abruptly. A day or two later we saw in the paper that a girl answering her description had taken her own life, and could not help wondering whether she were in trouble and seeking an abortion.

For a time we were licensed to handle narcotics but this proved to be a nuisance as well as a risk, for, as a veterinarian, I was believed (correctly) to be the holder of such large amounts of drugs as might be administered to a cow or a horse.

In those days we took our pay in all kinds of ways and were

glad to get it. One client who owed us a bill came in with a dressed hog. We paid him seven dollars, which he badly needed, canned the meat, and wrote the debt off. One day a client for whom we had done several jobs some time previously came in with a large box, which he set on the table. "Is the doctor in?" he asked Hazel. She told him I was out on a call.

"Tell him when he comes that this is for what I owe him," he said, and departed.

The box contained a dressed goat.

Although I was the first graduate veterinarian in a large area of the Panhandle and surrounding counties, we encountered a good many non-graduate practitioners, especially during our first years there. Some were out and out quacks, but a few did a fair job of their specialties, and we got along all right. One of these was a chap named Willie who campaigned for the state legislature as a veteran of World War I.

"Don't give me away," Willie confessed to me. "But I was inducted just two hours before the shooting stopped. I was on the train on my way to boot camp when we heard the news."

Willie was a great borrower. Having convinced the farmers in the area that horses' teeth needed going over at regular intervals, he did a brisk business in horse dentistry. After I arrived, he made use of several of my instruments on loan, including my speculum, an all but indispensible device for examining the mouths of horses and mules. When I passed a road construction camp one day and saw Willie muscling in on my territory with my tools, I resolved to reclaim the instruments.

It was a few weeks, however, before I was able to do so. I drove out to Willie's house one evening about sundown, but he was nowhere in evidence. Hearing a voice out back, I discovered a local M.D. with a considerable reputation for intemperance seated on a chopping block and entertaining himself by intoning poetry.

"Yes, Willie's in there," he told me cheerfully, gesturing toward the house. "I'm just waiting for him to die."

I found Willie in his bed. He did look bad all right, but he told me where the instruments were and made some excuse for not having returned them. A few days later I was dismayed to hear that he really had died that night. I doubt whether his doctor was much help in easing him out of the picture.

Willie was right in a way; there *was* something wrong with

the horses' teeth in that area. It may have been due to some vitamin lack or deficiency in the soil. Whatever it was, it gave me considerable experience in dentistry. Indeed, we had quite a lot of calls to doctor horses and mules for all kinds of ailments. On small ranches and farms, among hard-scrabble farmers who couldn't afford much in the way of motorized machinery, horses and mules were still widely used as work animals. In 1932, Dr. Heiser, the state veterinarian, had warned us to be on the lookout for sleeping sickness (encephalomyelitis), and we learned to watch for symptoms, the staggering gait, the seeming paralysis of the lips.

When a horse trader of sorts came driving a band of fifty head down the old Chisholm Trail toward Texas one day, he stopped and asked permission to hold the animals for a day or two of rest in the sale yard. Unable to make arrangements for this, he hunted out a rent pasture owned by Jack Farrier. The following day Jack called me. "There's something the matter with these horses, Doc," he said. "Maybe you'd better come out and have a look. One of them is staggering all over the place."

By the time I arrived, a second animal was staggering. Shortly, we noticed a third. We hastily hunted up the owner and, with his blessing, went over the entire herd. The disease appeared to be subclinical, but it was unmistakably encephalomyelitis. Several showed signs of being affected. I can tell you we were glad to see those animals move on out of the area.

After the drouth struck in earnest all over the Southwest every trace of the disease seemed to vanish. Later, we were to encounter a pretty bad epidemic in Nebraska, and still later, during the Sixties, we saw occasional cases among horses on the Nevada range. If the ailing horse could be kept on his feet, we found (we referred to this as "nursing"), he seemed to fare better and to have a better chance. A horse, like a man, is a peculiar animal in that, once down, he is too apt to give up. Then he is done for.

As epidemics too often do, the Nebraska bout resulted in a rush of drug claims and publications by unreliable firms. When the disease had somewhat subsided, government men were sent out to compile statistics on the number of animals treated, death loss, and recoveries. We were interested to learn that the percentage of recovery among the treated and the untreated proved about the same.

On Nevada ranches, we vaccinated a good many horses, making intradermal (between the layers of skin) injections at timed intervals, and felt they enjoyed considerable immunity for this reason. Of course we treated, too, because we felt obliged to take *some* measures and because it was expected of us. But, truthfully, we could not claim much effect.

The ideal as in all diseases of epidemic proportions was, of course, prevention, and occasionally a kind of light almost glimmered through the fog. In an area in South Dakota where horses were still in general use as work animals, around 1936, an epidemic of sleeping sickness sprang up at threshing time. In a spirit of watchfulness, all horses were temperatured each morning. If one showed the slightest reading, he was taken out and allowed to rest. Of the diagnosed cases, there occurred less than a twenty percent loss, and we thought we learned something from this practice. An observation concerning the number of victims that seemed to be weaned colts, gave rise to a theory that *suckling* colts just might enjoy a passive immunity from the milk of a mother that had suffered a light case. Such straws in the wind didn't help much. But they gave us something to cling to and served as conversation pieces for shop talk when we got together.

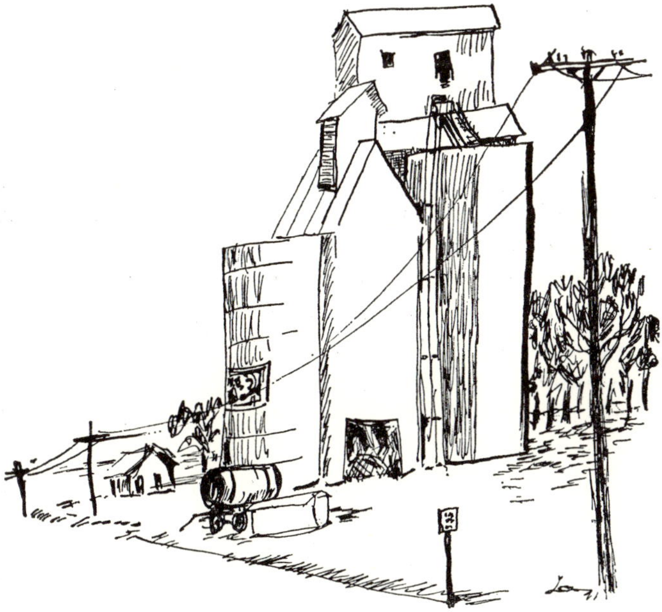

P.W.A. AND OTHER AILMENTS

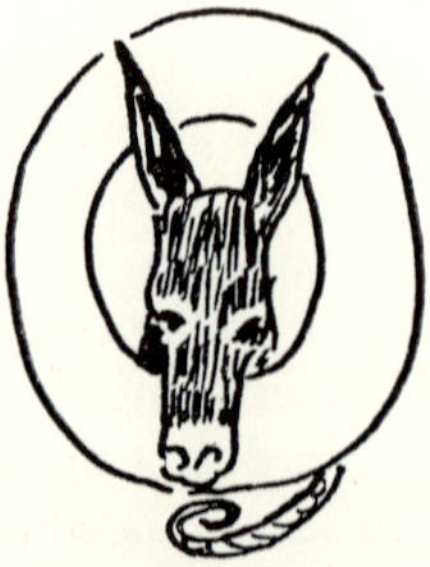

ONE PROJECT that gave us a good deal of work in the Panhandle was the highway grade built through sagebrush country during the drouth and Depression. The highway, to be a portion of a transcontinental road, was built by the Public Works Administration, known as the P.W.A. This is not to be confused with the Works Progress Administration, or W.P.A., which became the butt of so many jokes. The former was an unemployment project designed to help local areas. As did some other businesses, we enjoyed fringe benefits.

Hauling and grading was done largely by mule teams and contracts were let to private construction companies. Fifty percent of the labor hired by these companies had to be local. One of these outfits consisted of a gang of levee builders from Louisiana, and it was a real pleasure to watch those mule skinners at work. Four head of mules were hitched to each Fresno scraper and each skinner had to dump his own dirt. They all knew how to level and they were fast workers and had good mules. Almost literally, mountains of dirt were moved at a cost of eleven cents a yard. When they came into our area I was called out fairly frequently to doctor one or more of the mules, and I was glad to go.

One scrub outfit that gave me a little trouble was owned by a peculiar fellow who went by the name of Gunnysack Robinson. He had come by the name honestly, from his ingenuity in tying gunnysacks together to make traces for his mules. His skinners used a single crupper on the mules instead of breeching harness. To be sure, breeching harness was a kind of status symbol on farms when and where I grew up in southeast Kansas and I was almost grown before I saw my first set. But by the nineteen thirties and with a construction company, you expected something a little more modern than a simple crupper loop.

Robinson's mules were tough enough, but some of them were pretty ribby. When one of them came down with colic once, Robinson sent for me. "I reckon it might be just missmeal cramps he's got, Doc," he said frankly, "but I wanted to know." I allowed as how he was about right. I did quite a lot of work on the mules' teeth and Robinson ran up a good-sized bill. As are a horse's teeth, a mule's dentures are all in place when the animal is born; they just keep pushing up. Sometimes they have to be filed off or pulled out. Robinson kept saying he was too hard up to pay me. But I was hard up, too, and had a family to support.

Quite a few horse and mule sales were held around and I picked up some work inspecting animals to be shipped out of the state. When I heard about a mule that had sold for $125.00, a fair price for that time, I asked who had bought it. "Oh, some dirt mover around Buffalo," the sales manager told me. He riffled through his papers. "His name's Robinson."

"Well, we'll just attach that mule," I told him. "Robinson owes me a vet bill."

I didn't have long to wait. Gunnysack came around and paid the bill as though nothing had happened and we remained friends. That was just the way he operated.

Grading during that long hot summer was animal-killing as well as man-killing work. No horse could have stood up, but those mules did. Men and mules worked twelve hours a day. The mules had no noon meal, only a little water. A mule is a wonderful animal but something of a character, and it takes a character to handle him properly. You have to learn to think the way a mule thinks and then to out-think him. Sometimes that's not so easy.

One better-equipped outfit on the grade was run by a character named Honiker. Honiker drank a good deal and that sometimes caused trouble. But he had good mules and good harnesses and he took care of his animals. When he called one day to say his mules had been coughing for about six weeks I drove out to

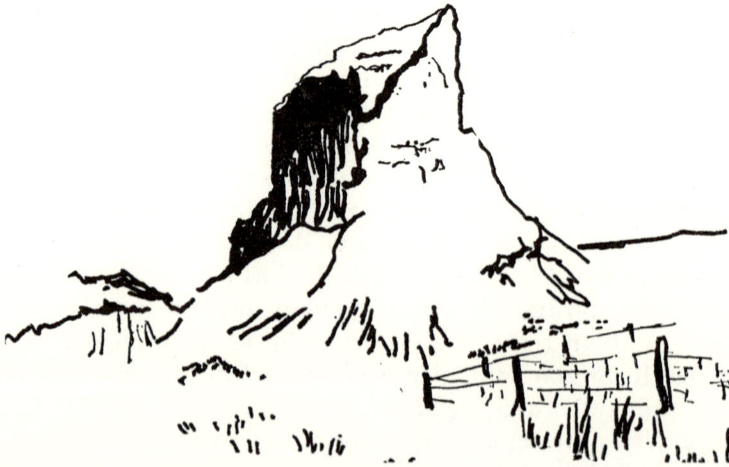

the camp. The mules were under the care of a "barn man," a fellow who wore a big black hat, flattened at the top and with a Bob Crosby crimp. His job was to throw up a moveable fence at each successive camp, to contain the animals, and to see that they were well fed and cared for. Honiker's mules were allowed to eat all they wanted when the day's work was finished. You can't do that with a horse. A horse will eat until he founders. But a mule has more sense.

As I approached Honiker's camp I could hear the mules coughing. I asked the barn man how late the crew worked.

"Well they stay out until dark drives them in," he told me. "On a clear day that's pretty late sometimes."

That Panhandle country gets as hot as blazes during the day, but it cools off quickly as nightfall approaches. In a lather when the temperature dropped, I reckoned, the mules were simply catching cold. "You tell Honiker to take the mules out of harness an hour before dusk," I said, "and let them cool off gradually. I don't think he'll have any more trouble."

I mixed up a beechwood creosote emulsion and instructed the barn man to give each animal a tablespoonful at prescribed intervals. He went up to the cook shack and came back with a bent tablespoon with a broken and wobbly handle. He would walk up to a mule, grab hold of its tongue with one hand, and jam the wobbly spoon into its mouth with the other. Of course the mule objected. The barn man employed all the cuss words he knew, but the emulsion went down somehow, and I stopped worrying.

With that heavy work and the weather we had that summer

the mules suffered constantly from galls. Honiker bought "Vicks Gall Cure" by the gallon. We made the cure (or a reasonable facsimile thereof) at home, from alcohol, methyl violet, tannic acid, and water. When Honiker moved his camp farther away we simply sent him the basic concoction and let him add the water.

One day he called me out to look at an aging mule with colic. "Do what you can for him," he told me. "He's no damn good, he's held back in the traces for ten years. But I don't want him groaning around the place."

"Honiker's just mad at that mule," the barn man told me. "He got up in the wagon this morning to give the mule an enema and the mule wasn't having any. He sent Honiker and the bucket ass over appetite."

I did what I could. But the next morning the mule was dead. "Honiker's mad at *us* now," the barn man greeted me. "He says it was you and me that killed that mule."

One of Honiker's skinners, a straw boss called Slim, phoned me one day to treat a stubborn case of sweeny, an atrophy or shrinking away of tissue caused by an injured nerve. The trouble may occur in others areas such as on the hip, but it's generally along the ridge of the scapula and may have been brought about by an ill-fitting collar, a prolonged side-draft pull, or by a too short doubletree. Partly for the sake of appearance, but chiefly to make the collar fit better, our method was to inject a mixture of chloroform and turpentine as an irritant to build up the shrunken area with connective tissue. Dean Dykstra of Kansas State had claimed the use of chloroform along with turpentine made the treatment less painful. Starting along the edge of the scapular ridge, we injected one and one-half cc's of the mixture at intervals of an inch or two at each site.

Reasoning in this case that I couldn't be making continual trips out, at Honiker's expense, to inject the one mule, I made fifteen injections of one and one-half cc's on either side. The tissue filled up all right. Indeed, it ballooned. I could only hope Honiker wouldn't see the mule until the swelling subsided. I had the report from Slim, who found the matter hilarious. "Honiker asked me what the hell happened to that mule. I told him we had that damned Price up here. You ought to have heard the names he called you." When the swelling went down the tissues had filled out all right and the mule looked fine. But I had learned a good lesson.

With our horses on the farm, sweeny was a fairly common

occurrence. The only treatment we or the neighbor knew then sounds a bit like witchcraft but it worked pretty well. We split the skin and inserted a dime as a counter irritant. Why a dime instead of a nickel or a penny? A silver dime was less apt to tarnish.

When Honiker had finished in our area he went on down to Oklahoma City and then started building grade out of Bethany. Once he called me in the middle of the night, drunk, to ask me to come down and doctor his pony, a distance of some one hundred and fifty miles. Of course I didn't go.

Honiker ran into a little trouble down there with a grocer who ran a small country store squarely in the middle of the scheduled grade, and who declined to move. Honiker humored the man for a time, built the grade up to the store and then went around to the other side. But one day he got sauced up and decided to fill the gap. Armed with a long pole, he went into the store and started knocking goods off shelves and tables and pitching cans and bottles and boxes down the aisles. The barn man took one look and ran for Honiker's wife. By then, the place was a mess and the grocer had called the sheriff. "Honiker's old lady put her head in through the door and said, 'Come on, Pop,' " my informer told me. "She and the barn man hustled Honiker into the car and set out, and crossed the county line two jumps ahead of the sheriff. The barn man went back and handed the grocer four hundred dollars to pay for the damages."

It was through one of these road grade crews that we had definite proof of the longevity of anthrax *(Bacillus anthracis),* a malignant, infectious ailment affecting animals, including man, and known as "ragpicker's" or "wool sorter's" disease. Anthrax spore has been known to withstand up to six hours of boiling. Whenever and wherever an outbreak occurred, the state veterinarian was obliged to map the area for posterity.

When the disease broke out in a herd of cattle in the vicinity of Waynoka, maps made thirty years previously revealed that a crew at work on a railroad grade in the vicinity had lost a number of horses to anthrax and had buried the animals at the site. At work on a grade to underpass (or to overpass) the railroad, a P.W.A. crew had unearthed the graveyard of bones, alive with anthrax spores. The cattle had chewed on the bones. We set to work to burn the remaining bones and to re-mark the site, which will stand as an anthrax area as long as records remain.

While testing for tuberculosis in Nebraska some years later,

I was privileged to work with the late Dr. L. Van Es, a medical doctor and researcher at the University of Nebraska with a considerable interest in the disease. As an experiment, Dr. Van Es sealed a bit of anthrax spores into a cornerstone at the university and then offered to bet a hundred dollars that the spores would still be alive at the end of one hundred years. So far as I know, he found no takers.

Dr. Van Es, a Hollander, was an authority on more than tuberculosis and anthrax. Whenever he talked at veterinarians' meetings, we all stayed awake and listened. I recall one session during which a mysterious soreness in lambs' eyes came under discussion. Ewes' eyes appeared unaffected by the ailment. After we had kicked this puzzle around for a time, Dr. Van Es arose.

"When I interned in human medicine, gentlemen," he told us, "we were taught to put silver nitrate into the eyes of newborn babies in order to ward off any infection the child might have incurred during the birth process. In my humble opinion, when you look into a ewe's *eyes* for the source of the trouble under discussion you are simply looking into the wrong end of the ewe."

One of my prize croppers had to do with a case I thought might be anthrax. Having overlooked nits in the ear of a cow that had died under suspicious clinical circumstances, I hastened to mail the ear in to the state lab with a request for a report. The nits hatched enroute. Had the disease proved to *be* anthrax, sufficient hosts would have been released to infect every animal in the state of Oklahoma, a veritable Pandora's box!

Once, on a small ranch near Mooreland, Oklahoma, I encountered another deadly member of the same family, malignant edema, a disease caused by a long-living, spore-forming organism introduced through a wound, in which tissues become supersaturated with body serum.

One bright fall morning a rancher called in considerable distress. He had found three or four dead calves among his herd of forty-one. Several other calves seemed to be swollen along the belly. I found the calves, big fellows in the neighborhood of two hundred and fifty to three hundred pounds, on a pretty, green rye patch. Several did, indeed, appear to have swollen bellies. As we drove the animals slowly toward the corral where I could examine them, two more keeled over. I knew that an animal with malignant edema rarely lived long enough to develop any kind of resistance, and, as we had no effective systemic bacterial drugs then, I could do little save clean out the wounds resulting from a recent castration and hope for the best. The owner assured me that a neighbor had treated the wounds following the operation.

I asked what had been used in the treatment.

"A mixture of some kind of machinery lubrication," the rancher told me, "with kerosene to keep the flies off and to guard against screw worms. I watched him and he was careful and clean. He put the mixture on with a brush."

When I asked to see the brush, the rancher looked puzzled. "I didn't think it would ever come clean so I threw it into the fire."

The toll came to twenty-one calves. I never found the source but there remained little doubt in my mind but that the spore had been somehow introduced on the bristles of that brush. Observing such cases, I came to wonder why we had not seen more of this kind of thing on the home farm during my boyhood. By our standards we were reasonably careful. We wiped the knife blade between jobs. But we used the same swab, dipped in a mixture of axle grease and turpentine, on calf after calf after calf. Actually, we were luckier than we ever knew.

We did lose a big mare colt to edema one autumn, the first of the disease I had ever seen. We had put her on the hayrake at haying time. When she developed a sore neck, we called in the local veterinarian, who diagnosed the trouble as "malignant edema." The following morning the mare was dead.

Relevant to our suspicion of the brush as a medium of culture is a chilling story one of my professors, Dr. Frick, used to tell in illustration of the sometimes ridiculous (in this case, fatal) extent of army spit and polish. When the members of a Veterinary Corps stationed at a given base began to lose to malignant edema almost every horse that for any reason underwent surgery, a school of veterinary medicine was called in to do some sleuthing. A young army private charged with keeping the surgical instruments clean and shining in their display case was habitually polishing the thoroughly sterilized tools with a lightly oiled rag, alive with edema spore.

POOR IN THE PANHANDLE

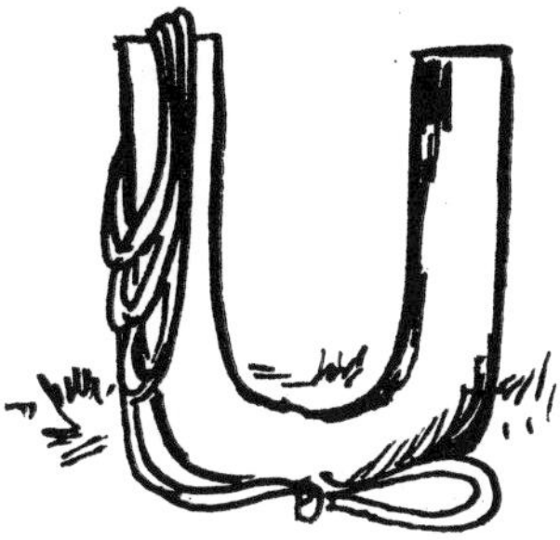

UNQUESTIONABLY, my most embarrassing moment occurred in the Panhandle in connection with milk fever. About the time the members of the veterinary profession thought they had an answer to milk fever, the solution was knocked into a cocked hat by some completely opposite circumstance. The assumption that depriving an animal of food helped to reverse the disease led to a premature conclusion that there was some connection somehow between the ailment and the cow's having plenty of green grass to make a milk supply.

One of our professors insisted that milk fever like some of our other short-sighted flapdoodles resulted from a demand that cows be bred to produce greater and greater quantities of milk. The cow might oblige, he said, but she was apt to break down in the process. "If the Lord had intended that a cow give sufficient milk to feed five *calves,*" he used to tell us, "He would have seen to it that she produced five calves at a dropping."

Because of a little run of good luck at treating the disease, I had grown pretty cocky about my own theories. Fortunately, the symptoms of milk fever are obvious. The animal moves with a staggering motion and turns her head to one side as though she has a kink in her neck. Her eyes have a glazed appearance. She may suffer paralysis, or even lapse into a coma as though her end were near. Presto, along comes the doctor with his pill bag. Following a simple calcium injection a cow that looked to be on her final trip might well get to her feet and walk away as though restored by some miraculous magic.

To be sure, I had no illusions about this being any kind of permanent panacea. Generally a heavy producer, as the professor had pointed out, the seemingly cured patient was apt to suffer recurring attacks of increasing severity at each successive parturition. I always advised the owner to get rid of the animal before the next gestation period following a second attack.

The cow in question belonged to a local M.D. who owned a farm in the vicinity. Impressed by two or three quick "cures" on my part, the good doctor had alerted the teacher of a high school class in vocational agriculture and suggested he bring his group to witness my next performance. Arriving in response to the doctor's call one day, I found teacher and students waiting and expectant.

I knew no qualms. Of such stuff, alas, is overconfidence. Following a briefing by the teacher, I stepped briskly forward, the center of an admiring audience. Kneeling beside the seemingly dying cow, I administered the injection. Arising, I moved back to await the anticipated resurrection. Turning her head to one side, the hapless cow emitted a deep sigh, closed her eyes, and quietly departed to meet her maker.

One phase of horse practice I especially disliked, saw a good deal of in the Panhandle, and never really learned much about, went by the broad name of "colic." Almost any bellyache thereabouts was diagnosed as "colic," a lay term that might cover a multitude of abdominal upsets involving pain. The source was too often obscure, the cure too often nebulous.

Both on the farm in Kansas and in the Panhandle, where the trees grew in profusion, the difficulty seemed to stem often from the animal's having eaten the leaves of the mulberry tree. For some reason a horse has a thing about mulberry leaves the way a cat has a thing about catnip, and the rough, coarse leaves and stems tend to form "birds' nests" in the large colon. Coarse alfalfa hay sometimes did the same, as did sagebrush when the animals fed on it because of dry weather.

Our usual treatment was with linseed oil administered by stomach tube. It was said, sometimes sarcastically, that the use of the stomach tube was Kansas State Veterinary School's single claim to fame. Truth or poetry, the technique we had learned there was sound and effective. An improperly inserted stomach tube causes medication to flow into the lungs, "drowning the horse (as the saying goes) on dry land." In the Wisner, Nebraska, area, where the expression still has a special significance, one practitioner habitually downgraded a competitor with whom he had feuded for some twenty years by declaring, "he drowned a horse on dry land."

Frequently, most especially on weekends, I was called upon to help out in some extracurricular and neighborly capacity, a good Southwest custom. One Sunday evening a request came for assistance in returning to the home ranch, some twenty-two miles distant, a band of mares the owner had brought into town as escort to colts consigned for shipping. "I hate to ask you on a Sunday and all, Doc," he told me. "But I need somebody who can *ride* to make the trip."

I told him, with secret relief, that I owned no mount.

"Oh, I've taken care of that," he said cheerfully. "You can ride Dobie." I knew the horse, a pretty stallion well known in the area. My human companion, it seemed, was to be a cowboy from the ranch, by the name of Dick.

Once started, the mares took off at full speed, reckoning, I suppose, that the colts were back at the ranch toward which they were headed. A prairie fire had recently gone through the range, burning the buffalo grass and sage to a charred mass, and the soot and ashes kicked up soon lost the galloping animals in an enveloping cloud. Coming, finally, to a drift fence, we were puzzled to find no trace of our charges.

"You ride one way and I'll go the other, Doc," Dick suggested. "One of us is bound to catch up with the buggers."

The sun set as I rode and darkness fell, but I neither came up with the mares nor found any aperture they might have negotiated. To spare the stallion, so played out he could hardly walk, I took turns riding and leading. In all that time I saw no sign of Dick. Nor did I have any notion of my own whereabouts until I came to the bank of the Canadian River. Beyond, in the far distance, I could see the dim lights of a ranch house. But I had learned by then not to be deceived by apparent nearness in that far flat country.

To add to my troubles, my gallant and handsome steed stood trembling and snorting on the bank and stubbornly declined to enter the water. I pulled and tugged and talked persuasively, finally employed all the cusswords in my repertoire. He took a few steps forward. But then, feeling the shifting sand underneath his feet, he went down. I had, almost literally, to carry him across the broad shallow channel.

Alternately walking and riding, I reached the ranch at two A.M., to find the homing mares lined up at the gate and watching our approach, my cowboy companion comfortably bedded in his bunk, and snoring lustily. The rancher's wife drove me back to Woodward in her Ford, an incredibly short journey.

One of the saddest (because usually unnecessary) conditions we encountered among the horses in the Panhandle was a disease of the feet called Laminitis brought on by overfeeding. Almost half the Shetland ponies we saw suffered from this ailment. I blamed the parents of the child owners. The first lesson a youngster should be taught when he is given a horse as a gift is not to be constantly offering the animal sugar lumps and anything else he will eat. We always advised prospective horse buyers to take a good hard look at the feet of any animals they were about to be purchasing. If a horse shows distinct rings about his hooves he should be rejected, or, at least, suspected. The overfeeding of oats is somewhat less dangerous than the overfeeding of wheat or rye, since oats contain more fiber, which aids digestion.

Once it was believed that if you withheld water from a foundered horse you might prevent the onslaught of the disease. We achieved pretty good results by the simple method of digging a shallow trench, filling it with four or five inches of water, and tying the animal in such a way that he was forced to stand in the puddle. This decreased circulation to the feet by keeping the feet cool. This was an old-fashioned remedy, but we never found a drug equal in therapeutic value to this method.

I once rode a horse that belonged to Tom Mix. This momentous event occurred on the Davidson Ranch south of Arnett, Oklahoma, in the vicinity of the Packsaddle Bridge across the South Canadian River. When the famous 101 Ranch Circus went broke in Washington, D.C., Zack Miller of the 101 had Mix under contract. Sensing no doubt that the circus was tottering, Mix had resigned a bit earlier, allegedly violating his agreement. Zack sued and won. Somehow in the legal settlement, he came by the horse, which wound up on the ranch owned by his friend Davidson.

We had been scheduled to test cows on the range. But, then, Davidson had asked that we hold off until round-up time in order to save the cowboys work. As a reward for our cooperation he invited us to a dinner of wild turkey and roast buffalo, a specialty of the ranch. As a special dispensation, I was invited to go for a canter on Tom Mix's horse, which knelt for me to mount, just as in the pictures.

When I undertook to assist the cowboys in the separation of the buffalo calves (to be sold the following day) from their mothers, I learned a thing or two about buffalo. Unlike domestic calves of the genus *Bos,* a young buffalo fails to give warning by facial expression when he is about to charge.

On the following day I went briefly into the buffalo business by bidding in seventeen of the calves. There again I made a miscalculation. A fence that will nicely contain a domestic calf is a paper tiger to a buffalo. We sold the calves to a butcher in Oklahoma City who wanted them for his Christmas trade.

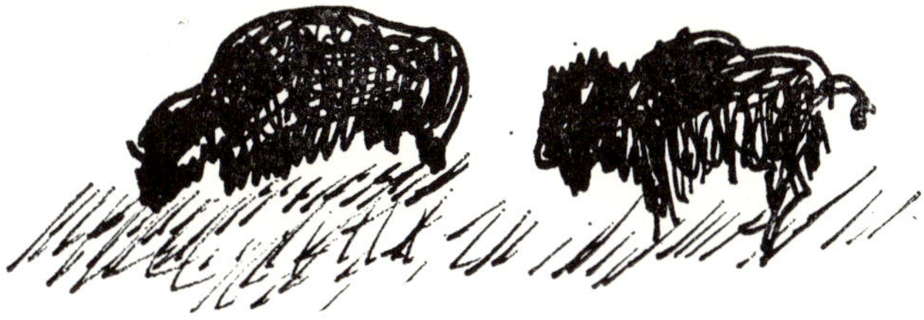

It is interesting to note how the Packsaddle Bridge came by its name. Sent to the South Canadian to quiet an Indian uprising, General George Custer drove his wagon train into the river ford, only to be attacked by a band of Indians concealed in tall grass along the banks. Hastily abandoning the train, the intrepid Custer was obliged to sacrifice pack animals, saddles, wagons, and equipment. According to local ranchers, the rims of buried wheels could still be seen in the soft deep sand of the riverbed in the vicinity of the bridge when the stream dried away each summer.

I like to say, too, that I once rode a famous rodeo mount that performed in Tex Austin's group. Invited to England for a series of appearances, one of Tex's boys, Rusty Corwin, left his horse with us over a weekend so that I could check it out for glanders, a requirement for all of the animals scheduled to make the trip. In order to ride with Austin's crack team, a cowboy must have placed first, second, or third in a recognized rodeo.

The horses Austin took to England were all beautiful, well-trained animals, and Rusty's was no exception.

The trip, however, proved something of a fiasco. Corwin told me his version of the story after the troop returned to this country. Having heard that rodeo was a rough game in which animals were sometimes maimed and killed, a British humane organization succeeded in getting regulations passed that (according to Corwin) "took the sport right out of the show." The public stayed away in droves. One rule in particular prohibited the use of the "rowel spur," substituting a small knobby army spur in its stead. Artificial means to induce bucking were also taboo. In the Southwest, cowboys who rode bucking horses made use of a "flank rope," generally a length of sash cord tied around the flank. The new regulations also required that calves be roped with a breakaway loop instead of being thrown and tied.

Some of these rules later broke over into Canadian performances, and in the name of humanity some of them were certainly justified. But Southwestern cowboys generally took a dim view and Southwestern rodeos remained pretty rough. Still, some of them were great to watch because of the skill of both horses and the men who rode them as though man and animal were one and inseparable. In steer bulldogging, for example, when the rider threw the rope in an attempt to catch the steer by the horns, the horse turned on a dead run at a forty-five-degree angle the moment the rope left the rider's hands.

To be sure, for all its beauty of precision, the performance sometimes had a sad aftermath. The steer might well roll end over end, his horns shelled off or his neck broken. Bands of Indians followed the shows in order to salvage the meat of the victims. Chuckwagon races (famous in Canada), on the other hand, were more dangerous for *men* than for the animals involved, so no *humane* society protested. Panhandle rodeos always included steer roping. Horses that took part in calf roping were schooled in a different manner.

To an old-time cowboy who has participated in (or even witnessed) cutting and roping horses at work and in the ring, where their mettle is matched against that of other working stock, the present-day rodeo put on primarily for show and secondly for skill has a phony aspect. Just as the Brahma steer is not only raised for meat but for his performance in the ring, the bucking horse is no longer a half-broken animal, but one *raised* to buck for his supper. Presently, all animals that perform in a given rodeo may come from the selfsame "ranch," a training ground devoted to rearing props for the professional cowboy who flies from show to show to entertain his public, a performer who may never have *seen* a working roundup, let alone taken part in this essential function.

To watch a cutting horse at work in the show ring is a thrilling experience. As any cowpoke knows, the first lesson his horse must learn is to get a proper lead on the steer he is about to cut out of the herd. Instinctively, or reminded by a touch from his rider, a trained cutting horse will always lead with the inside leg. In calf roping, horses learn quickly to stop the moment the rope settles, so that the rider can peel off and throw the calf. In steer roping, as I have said, the horse turns at a forty-five-degree angle and keeps going.

The skill called "dogging" can be taught to almost any good saddle horse. The rider dismounts from the running horse, which has been trained to get out of the way, and wrestles the steer to the ground. I have seen cowboys throw a steer in as little as seven seconds. Individual differences in steers could, it seemed to me, make a contest sometimes unfair. The bulldogger might, for instance, draw a "rubberneck" requiring up to thirty seconds for throwing, and so put on a more spectacular performance than a dogger with equal or greater skill at the game.

The Panhandle cowboys as we knew them were a rugged lot, who had literally grown up in the saddle. As young boys they had learned to ride and to rope because the knowledge was taken for granted. I recall a story told by one of these that demonstrates toughness as well as ingenuity. I cannot of course vouch for the truth of the narration.

Because that was his name, I will call the cowboy Combs. As range riders, Combs and the other cowpokes were under orders to castrate on the spot any scrub bull encountered during their tour of duty, and they carried knives for the purpose. Coming across one such animal on a hot day, Combs related, he roped and tied the animal and proceeded with the operation.

"I reckon I'd cut half a hundred of his caliber in my time, and without any sweat. But this one gave a sudden lunge when

I was only half through and knocked the knife out of my hand into the tall buffalo grass. I never did find that knife. Hot as it was, I didn't dare leave the job unfinished. So I just got down and used my teeth on the bugger."

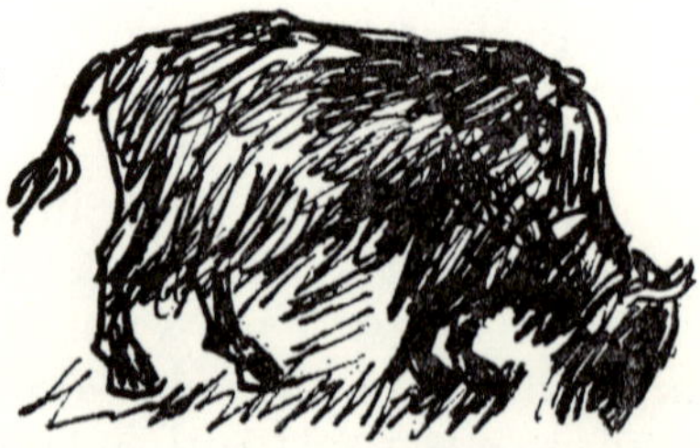

DUST

HAD WE NOT LIVED and worked in the Panhandle during the dustbowl era of the Thirties, I scarcely would have credited the millions of descriptive words written about that catastrophic time. Easterners, unsympathetic and beyond an understanding of the buying and killing program resulting from the drouth, were quick to lay blame for the debacle on the farmers and ranchers of the area. To be sure, if the prairie sod had never been broken there might never have been a dustbowl. But neither would the killing have been necessary had the country been blessed those years with anything like normal rainfall for grass and crops.

The drouth set in following several years of declining market prices for crops and livestock. Generally a farmer-stockman can weather bad years, being a gambler by disposition with both weather and the vagaries of market ebb and flow. But this was a prolonged combination of bad luck in both commodities. During years of drouth and low prices, stock owners had held off in the vain hope of up-turn. As a result herds had multiplied to the place where ranges were over-grazed and over-populated.

Having invented the phrase, "Man went too far west with the plow," writers used it over and over to describe the situation. It appeared that man had also gone too far west with the *cow*. But this was hindsight. Certainly no less than an oracle could have foreseen the devastating mixture of drouth and depression that beset these plainsmen and their families. These were years of misery for both men and animals. We came to marvel at the hardly believable endurance of both.

The trouble did not arise from a single year, but from season after season of scant rainfall. So long as there was sufficient rain to nourish vegetation, both native and planted, to keep the soil in place, the wind, which blows strongly throughout the Southwest, was no obstacle. The percentage of families that deserted their homes and holdings when the dust was whipped up to cloud proportions, burying fences and even houses underneath tons of soil, was not great. These were only the families that were interviewed and photographed again and again, and written about. Most farmers toughed it out. This portion of the Southwest had been settled by men and women who liked open prairie with its endless vista and its solitary expanse. And even through the worst of the dust most kept faith that the grass would come back, that the land would bloom again.

Their faith was justified, the grass did come back. But those were hard years, with marginal living conditions for both rural and townspeople. I recall a stop one morning in the town of Supply for a bite of breakfast at a small cafe. When I handed the proprietor a five dollar bill to pay my modest charge, she said, "I'm sorry, Sir, I have no change. Just pay me the next time you're through."

"I'll cash it across the street," I offered.

She shook her head. "*He* wouldn't have change either," she told me. "Nobody in this town would have change for a five these days. Just pay me the next time you stop. We're all in the same boat you know."

After a while we became more or less accustomed to the dust. I won't say we learned to like it or even to ignore the clouds of dirt. But we learned a little about how to live with them and survive. Even in the more tightly built houses (of which ours was not one) there was no escape. With windows closed and rags stuffed into the cracks, dust still piled up around the legs of the chairs and tables and lay in drifts across the bedding. We became inured to the taste of grit in our food, and forgot the smell of clean air in our nostrils.

We heard and read of deaths attributed directly to the dust. I expect these came to more than we knew about. I know there were deaths farther north (in western Kansas) that resulted from people becoming lost in weather too cold for survival. I have always felt that the high incidence of emphysema that came up later could probably have been traced directly to the fact that people went for months at a time without drawing a breath of clean air into their lungs.

When the wind changed, dust arose, within moments, so thick you could hardly, literally, see your hand before your face. The sun might come up, the day seem comparatively clear, at six o'clock. By eight it would be as dark as night, the entire countryside enveloped in rolling clouds of choking topsoil. Travelers declared, truthfully, that they were unable to see their own radiator caps. I never worried about this so much. When I looked down and failed to see the earth beneath my feet, I felt lost indeed.

But men and women had to go on with their work and with their lives. This was not, as a tornado would have been, a temporary disruption from which they could seek shelter. We kept moistened sponges tied over our mouths and nostrils day after day as we went about our assignments. When the sponges became saturated with mud we washed them out with water from the canvas bags we always carried lashed to the bumpers of our vehicles, and put them on again. The air was so filled with static electricity originating from the bombardment of dust particles that most cars had to be grounded by a length of chain. The one exception I knew was the Model T, which had a unique electrical system. More than once when a windmill was turned on I saw sparks jump as much as six inches from the mechanism.

People made jokes about the dust, even in the midst of it. Asked, "How's *your* wheat look, Joe," a farmer is said to have replied, "Looked fine as it passed the house. You'll have to ask the fellow where it landed."

Dust piled up in drifts like snow, miniature sand dunes in a constant state of locomotion. Dust formed in humps and hillocks behind clumps of sagebrush and mesquite and dead Russian thistles, termed tumbleweeds because of their proclivity for breaking loose and rolling for miles before the wind, to bank up against some fence or building. When the wind changed, the drifted dust swirled back into the air and was off again in a new direction. When an occasional light rain fell through the blowing motes, the drops descended as mud. Even on "clear" days the sun remained invisible.

People slept with their faces swathed in wet towels. Schools closed, for days sometimes, because of the danger of children becoming lost on the roads. If the dust thickened toward closing time, pupils were kept at the schoolhouse overnight, where stocks of food and blankets were kept. We heard about a traveling salesman who drove, one unusually nasty day, into the town of Boise, Oklahoma.

"How far is it to Guymon?" he grumbled.

"About sixty miles," the service station attendant informed him.

"How far to Clayton, New Mexico?"

"About the same."

"Liberal, Kansas?"

"Likewise. I reckon it's about sixty miles to any place you could ask about, Mister."

"You're wrong," the salesman said grimly, peering into the wall of dust. "It's not more than twenty feet to hell from right here."

Having driven out on a call once, I lost my bearings and came to a dead stop. The wind that day was blowing fitfully and hard, first in one direction and then in another. For a time I would be enveloped in a dense cloud and then the air would clear sufficiently for me to see, however dimly, a few telephone poles ahead along the roadside. I sat for minutes as though in a bottle of milk, or dirty water. When the cloud lifted for a bit I saw that I had stopped squarely in the middle of an intersection of two cross-state highways.

Carried by south and west winds, the dust moved north and east, to blanket the Flint Hills, the Ozarks, the Osages. Nebraska relatives wrote that they awoke one morning to find their porches covered with reddish residue from the Panhandle.

When sufficient rain came, finally, the drifts crusted over and hardened. Men and animals walked over the tops of buried fences in a strange unfamiliar landscape. In many cases, only the taller structures, such as windmills and silos and elevators stood above the ruin. You might drive for miles upon end without seeing a sign of green. I remember one unforgettable sight. A small house, half-buried but still inhabited, boasted a line of blossoming geraniums on an inside windowsill.

I also recall two lines from a poem written by a Blackwell attorney, Roy Cox, who rode through the area on a train and scribbled the verses on an envelope:

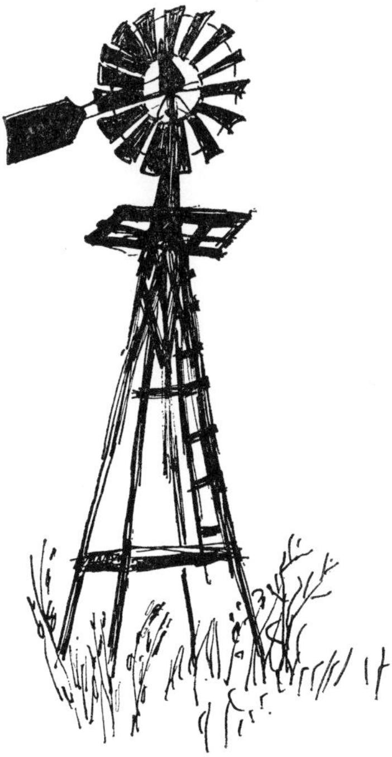

"Everything's gone but the windmill,
And it would go if it could."

Following the debacle, you heard the phrases, "blowed-on fields," and "blowed-off fields," the former to describe areas where dust had settled in mounds to harden over whatever vegetation had been left standing. Because of these humps and hummocks, "blowed-on fields" were more difficult to reclaim. The "blowed-off" fields at least possessed the virtue of being level for cultivation.

In June of 1934 I accepted a job with the Federal Veterinary Force of the Bureau of Animal Industry, at a salary of $1,800.00 per annum; my assignment, then, to test for tuberculosis throughout the state. Along with most of the farmers and ranchers upon whom we were dependent, we were just about down to bedrock. Our clients did well to eke out a subsistence for themselves and their families. Few had the means to buy feed for their animals, let alone to hire a veterinarian for their care. With wheat selling for twenty-five cents a bushel and cattle proportionately low, even a doctor's or a dentist's fee was a luxury.

In August I was taken off tuberculosis testing and set to work on the appraising, buying, and killing program. The program had begun to the west of us in New Mexico and Arizona. A B.A.I. supervisor who stopped in Woodward that summer told of seeing as many as 10,000 dead cattle piled up around a dry Arizona waterhole; half-starved animals lacking the strength to travel to the next pond or windmill. In our own area the cattle population was out of hand. Ponds had gone dry and little save Russian thistle and sagebrush was left upon which an animal could graze, and these were for the most part buried under tons of dust.

Later, buying and killing quotas were set up in Kansas for cattle and in Nebraska, almost equally hard-hit, for hogs.

I was only one veterinarian among the seventy-five or so engaged in this horrendous work around the state. For two or three years no rain of measurable proportion had fallen on the parched land. Ranchers and farmers were in dire need of the pittance the animals would bring. Our orders were spelled out. When processing space was available and livestock strong enough to make the nearest shipping point, we bought "live" and were more than happy to do this. Often, as in the case of the all-black town, we had no live quota. Slaughterhouses were glutted, feed and water supplies for the animals were exhausted. All had to go.

For most of the time the young Indian traveled with me to do the sticking, and so I was spared that. However he felt about the job, he was prompt and proficient. As with me, it was a living for himself and his family. We were also given specific instructions for selecting and appraising the animals' worth and for compensating the owner. I was assigned two helpers, generally local ranchers chosen by the Extension department for their ability to appraise. Quotas for buying both live animals (fit to be shipped to packing houses) and those doomed to be shot were set according to their condition and to available facilities for shipping, canning, or processing the meat. We were notified by wire each week as to the number of dead and the number of live animals we were to buy in a given area. We were judge and jury as well as executioner. The choice in each case was left up to us.

Animals in each group were classified according to age as calves, yearlings, and mature. We had a low and a high price allowable for each live animal purchased and we tried to give the owner the high range when we could. A live cow was appraised anywhere from thirteen to twenty dollars. We could go as high as sixteen dollars for a yearling or as low as eight. A calf might bring anywhere from four to eight.

We also had a leeway for group classification. We could classify an eight-month-old as a yearling, and frequently did. Or we could label a twelve-month-old "mature." Generally a yearling was anything under two. Prices for dead animals (those obviously unfit for meat or for which no packing facilities were available) were set and standard. A dead calf was worth four dollars, a yearling eight dollars, a mature animal twelve dollars. An animal sentenced to be shot was so labeled; there could be no mistake.

The owner was allowed to keep one live-purchased animal of his choice for meat. The rest were shipped from the closest shipping point to the nearest available slaughterhouse or cannery. Some weeks our quota consisted of four hundred live and eight hundred dead. Some weeks we had no live quota at all.

Contrary to stories told outside the area, we had no difficulty with owners. No man wants to see his animals die of starvation, and the subsidy paid was desperately needed. A few days without food or water made an animal "unfit." Frequently owners called and begged us to come. Most of them were without feed. Many were without water, even for their own use. As little as it seemed, the government paid more for animals than they would have brought on a saturated market. Invariably, more animals were offered for sale than we had instructions to buy. If rain fell in one area of the state, the quota for that area was quickly cut. People lived, but hardly thrived, on hope.

We always screened the premises. If we found water in fair supply and the cattle chewing their cuds, we tried to talk the owners into hanging on for a while. We called meetings in schoolhouses and at Grange halls to explain the program. Occasionally we received a call from Wichita or from some other packing center asking us to kill closer. Too many cattle were being found dead in railroad cars, having died en route of malnutrition. Animals driven a considerable distance to railroad stockyards sometimes fell dead on the road or in the holding pens.

Slaughtering animals as we did must have appeared both heartless and wasteful to those who were shocked by headlines out of the Southwest. I know that in the East we had a bad press. But those outside the area could hardly visualize existing conditions. We encountered families with both wells and ponds dry and no water available within a twenty-mile radius. Water was hauled, often by mule wagon, for house use and to water chickens, horses, and hogs. Gardens planted in the spring of 1934 did not come up until the spring of 1935, and promptly died for want of moisture.

Wherever we went we were followed by groups of men and women bent on salvage of the hardly salvageable. We referred to these as "meat hounds" or "hide hounds" and left them alone. They lived a nomad, marginal existence, going from place to place like gypsies. Smoke curled up from their fires, built among the slaughtered animals. They moved about, cooking, drinking coffee, skinning carcasses for the hides, and slashing away at the blue, unappetizing meat.

Once on my rounds I came across a family camped in the middle of a dry arroyo, where their ancient car had given up the ghost. Even the pistons had been set out on the dusty ground. I felt obliged to warn them that in case of a flash flood resulting from a cloudburst up the arroyo they would be in a precarious position. More than one party of unwary campers, stopped for shelter in such a dry watercourse in that country, have been swept to their deaths by an unexpected deluge.

"Bone hounds" gathered up bleached skeletons to be made into fertilizer. Tatterdemalion and pathetic as these followers were, they had their merit, as did the coyotes, the eagles, and the turkey buzzards that fed on the meager flesh. Otherwise, farmers would have been obliged to burn or to bury the animals in the stone-hard earth. The visits I came to dread most were to small family farms where cows and calves were family pets. I recall especially a trip into red hill country north of Woodward to kill an old Jersey whose milk had nourished the sorrowing children. I felt like a murderer. But the cow was long since dry, her feed bin empty, and the family needed the pittance she would bring.

Occasionally something humorous happened, a good thing. On one farm in Muskogee County a heavy stand of timber grew behind the farmhouse. The cattle were in an open field. When I fired the first shot I heard a scream that scared me half out of my wits. "That's just my wife," the farmer assured me. "She's gun-shy. Carries on like that every time she hears a gun fire."

Each time I shot the scream was repeated, but at each shot the sound seemed to come fainter and farther away. Presently I could no longer hear it.

"I reckon you'll have to pay me for the wife, too," the farmer observed dryly when the time came to settle up. "She seems to have taken off for tall timber."

If the animals were mortgaged, which they often were, we had to obtain a signed release from the mortgage holder. But the rule held that the owner retained sixty percent of the selling price. Sometimes the mortgagee brought pressure on the owner to take less than his allowable, or accepted his forty percent and took a further mortgage on hogs, turkeys, chickens, ducks, or whatever the farmer had left. Most bankers took their allotted share and wrote the debt off. Most bankers gave us blanket leeway to appraise, too, and we appreciated their trust.

We did, however, have one amusing encounter with an appraiser sent out by a Federal Land Bank to double check our figures. We had gone out to buy cattle from an ornery rancher with a herd of wild Ayreshires. I'll call the rancher Ayres. One of my own appraisers, Harry Blaisdell, had ridden for the Big-V Ranch at the same time Ayres had ridden for the rival 101 so no love was lost between the two men. The land bank held a mortgage on Ayres' animals all right. But the bachelor who owned the dry pasture also had a rent bill against them and wanted his share.

Apprised of the second creditor, the land bank man set out to drive the thirty miles back to town to learn whether the cattle could be sold without payment of the pasture bill, and left us to cool our heels and to try to hold the cattle (if we could) in a flimsy, wire-fenced corral until his return with the verdict. Whenever we approached the enclosure, those wild-eyed "coyotes" stampeded and hit the fence on the opposite side. When the cowboys rode around that way the animals surged toward us. Two more mass surges and the entire herd broke through the fence and set off across the prairie in a cloud of dust, scattering wire and posts as they went.

Having waited around without food until well after noon we packed up our gear and departed. Around fifteen miles down the road we saw our man lurching and weaving toward us in his V-8. It was easy to see where he had spent the morning. Coming abreast, he stopped and threw out a gunny sack filled with shaved ice and three-two beer. He neither mentioned the grass bill nor inquired about the Ayreshires, long since departed in search of greener pasture. If they were ever rounded up again they were checked out by another crew.

One day we drove out to a big ranch owned by a man known as Fewclothes Selman, who had ridden the Chisholm Trail as a young buck. Owning nothing during his Chisholm days save his horse and the clothes on his back, he had come by the nickname, which had stuck. Selman was a cowhand of the old school, a skilled saddleman and roper, and a good friend to everyone he encountered. His cattle were in better shape than most and we had a considerable live quota. Of the seven or eight hundred head inspected, we culled only ninety. The rest were to be shipped from the nearest shipping point, the town of Quinlan, a hamlet of some one hundred and fifty people, twenty to thirty miles distant. We agreed to meet Selman there to take a stockyard count of the animals.

Sensing, correctly, that there might be a shortage of holding pens, Selman started the drive four or five hours before daylight broke. When we reached Quinlan about mid-morning we found all of the pens full and the town teeming with bawling cattle, dust, cowpokes, and aroused townspeople armed with brooms and mops in an effort to protect their premises.

During the count my attention was briefly distracted by a small boy seated on a top rail who kept saying, "That's *our* cow in there." But in the press of the morning's work I forgot him.

Shortly after the twenty stock cars filled with animals had pulled out I heard the kid again. "That was *our* cow in there," he insisted. This time I listened.

"Where's your Dad?" I asked uneasily.

"He's back yonder at our house."

"Could you bring him here?"

"The kid knows our cow all right," the father told us. "Two big herds went by early this morning and I've not seen her since."

I followed the only possible procedure. I wired ahead and had the train stopped at Waynoka for a search of the cars. Sure enough the missing cow was aboard. I was obliged to hire a truck to haul her back to Quinlan.

That was another day we went without eating. By the time the mixup was straightened out the only cafe in town had long since run out of food and closed its doors. After considerable search, someone dredged up a pint fruit jar of questionable gin, which served us as breakfast, lunch, and dinner.

On windy days, rolling tumbleweeds presented a considerable road hazard. A light car in high gear hit by a mess of tumbleweeds will almost veer off the roadway. One day I heard about another Chisholm Trail rider, from Dobie Springs, by the name of Sweet, who was driving along his line fence one breezy evening in his pickup, when so many tumbleweeds collected underneath his chassis that the car stalled. Sweet was never able to explain what possessed him to light a match in order to see what he was doing. The oily thistles caught, burned the four tires off his pickup, and took all the fence posts from around his cattle corral.

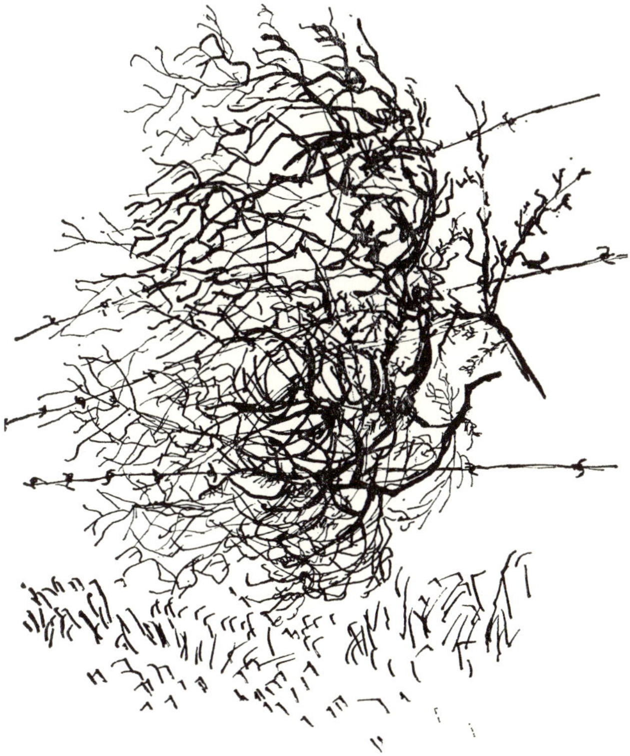

Even after the rains came and the grass grew back, ranges were still over-populated and grazing remained subnormal for a long time. In an effort to tide the farmers over and to keep breeding stock alive, a plan was instituted for the shipment of feed in from the outside. I don't know what moves some people to think it's all right to cheat the government, but too often this feed was inedible when it arrived. I recall especially one shipment of baled cornstalks. Devoid of leaves, or even husks, the stalks would have been of little value in *good* condition. These had been baled wet and were saturated with mold. We condemned two hundred tons of the stuff and gave the stalks to the farmers to stop washes in their fields.

When the rains began, the western prairie grass came back more rapidly than did the timber grass in the eastern part of the state. When word came that a surplus of unpastured Johnson grass existed in Louisiana levee country, the B.A.I. shipped many trainloads of cattle there in the hope that the animals might be kept alive until sufficient rain fell in the Dustbowl to bring the range grass back. An R (for rehabilitation) was branded on the hip of each animal shipped. For this reason they were generally referred to as "Roosevelt cattle."

The project proved a bit of a fiasco. When roundup time came it was discovered that many of the animals had disappeared. We could only guess they had found their way into Cajun pots. But thanks to the tuberculosis testing which was resumed as soon as the buying was finished, the survivors were at least brought back into an area practically free of that disease.

TUBERCULOSIS

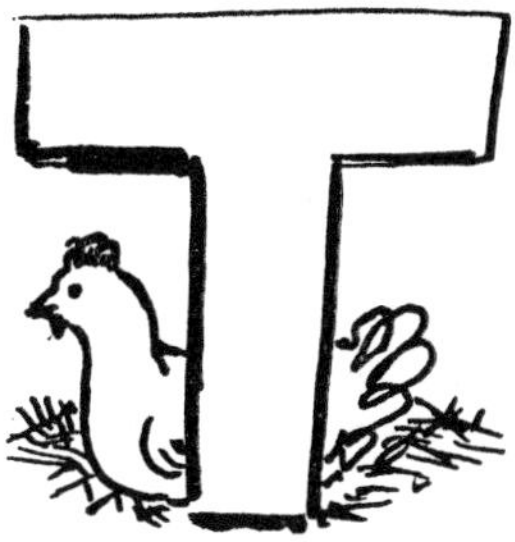

THE FIRST WORK of the Bureau of Animal Industry, established in 1883, was with pleural pneumonia in cattle. By the turn of the century Texas fever had been all but brought under control. Tuberculosis, brucellosis, and hog cholera programs came later. Although I admit that my opinion may be colored by the fact that I worked so long with tuberculosis, I think this was the greatest piece of work done by the B.A.I. Tuberculosis in an animal, as is cancer in a man, is an insidious disease. An entire herd can become infected before an owner, or even an expert, is aware. I had worked from June until August 1934 at tuberculosis testing and I went back to it with enormous relief when the buying and killing was done.

As mapped by the B.A.I., animal tuberculosis showed a distinct and interesting pattern of distribution. In the eastern part of the United States, animals were crowded together as in dairy herds, and incidence was heavy. Toward the west where animals were more scattered we saw far less tuberculosis. Inspectors in the packing houses and testers in the field enjoyed good cooperation, which accounts in large part, I am sure, for the success of the enterprise. Tubercular lesions are comparatively easy to detect in the slaughterhouse, and men in the field were prompt with follow-up into the herd from which the animals came.

Chronic diseases, such as tuberculosis, Texas fever, and

brucellosis have always been best controlled on an area basis, and that is what the bureau tried to do. Very little control work had been done prior to the Depression but much was done during it. Probably this was one of the few good things that came out of this trying time because men were available to do research and field work. When the program was started in earnest a great deal was accomplished in a brief span of years. Because of milk and dairy ordinances, the work began properly in eastern cities, and moved west. The discovery had been made that most tuberculosis in humans came as a result of bovine tuberculosis. As a boy I can remember seeing many "hunch-backed" people. I know now that these were more than likely tubercular. Fortunately hunch-backed people have almost disappeared from the streets.

Our method was to inject the animals with tuberculin and go back in 72 hours to read any reaction. I spent Monday, Tuesday, and Wednesday driving about to farms and ranches to make injections. On Thursday, Friday, and Saturday I covered the same territory, to check results. Although it wasn't according to the book, I did a little private practice in the evenings, and quite a bit on Sunday. Certainly I wasn't taking anything from any other veterinarian's pocket, for there were none in the area. As a matter of fact, I myself took little pocket money. But I had client-friends still dependent upon my services.

As a fringe benefit of tuberculosis testing, we came across some interesting facts concerning the spread of the disease. Sometimes we made ourselves pretty unpopular. One better-known ranch in Oklahoma raised and sold fine Shorthorns as breeding stock. I will call the ranch Bar-X. Farmers and stockmen had come to point with considerable pride to cows serviced by Bar-X bulls. When we started coming up with a heavy percentage of reactors in these farmers' herds, we began a little sleuthing.

Approximately one-third of the Bar-X herd proved to be infected with tuberculosis! Through these elegant bulls the disease was being spread throughout the state and beyond state borders. This discovery resulted in quite a bit of embarrassment, but it also was responsible for a considerable mop-up of a prime tuberculosis source.

We also made a discovery in the so-called "milking parlors," an innovation of the time. Each parlor held four cows, which were brought in relays at milking time and fastened in stanchions. When the four had been milked, they were taken out, the feed buckets were refilled, and a second foursome brought in. Thus the second four partook of the first quartet's slobbers, and any bacteria their predecessors had left. We found many parlor reactors before we got onto that one.

Reactors proved so frequent in dairy herds shipped from Wisconsin that we came to suspect, finally, that unscrupulous buyers were purchasing reactor cows there and shipping them in to sell at auction. Inasmuch as tuberculosis is readily transmittable to humans through milk, this was, if true, a criminal practice.

In eastern Oklahoma counties, with no herd laws and few corrals, we were obliged to serve often as cowhands as well as testers, roping, tying, and sometimes even rounding up animals prior to injection and again for reading. A local editor, we learned, had recently incurred the displeasure of many of the natives by editorializing for fences and herd laws in the area. Aside from a reluctance on the part of a farmer to go to the work of building fences, I have never quite understood the stubborn resistance to herd laws. But resenting regulations just seems to be a natural reaction. Where we worked in Nevada, eighty percent of the land was publicly owned under the Bureau of Land Management and range was open. But that is big country, with less risk of mingling and crossbreeding.

We ran across some rugged individuals in those eastern Oklahoma hills. During my drives about the countryside I had frequently passed a small country schoolhouse in a picturesque setting, a kind of landmark for a stranger. Riding by one morning accompanied by my guide, who happened to be the local sheriff, I was startled to see that all that remained of the building was a bed of smouldering ashes.

"Burned down last night," the sheriff said. "But we've got a pretty good lead. Old K down the road has a daughter who taught there last winter. Board fired her this spring. Several hereabouts heard old K swear that if she couldn't teach there nobody else was a-going to."

Most of the farmers in that area were pretty casual about their stock. Rounding up cattle one day for a test I came across a dead hog that had obviously died of cholera and hunted up the owner in a hurry.

"That so?" he drawled. "Well, now, I've been seeing dead hogs around these woods for quite some spell. That must be what they're dying of."

Occasionally we ran into trouble with reservation Indians

who would butcher a cow following an injection for fear she would come up a reactor. With a cow here and a cow there, all to be rounded up, work went at a snail's pace, until someone smarter than the rest of us thought up a wonderful scheme to facilitate the roundup. WPA employees, fairly plentiful in the area, were set to work building a big corral and chute in the approximate center of the county. When the corral was ready, we called a meeting, elected a boss man, and named a testing day. Farmers were invited to the big testing "perlew" and asked to bring along all their cattle.

The scheme worked. These were sociable folks who loved a get-together of whatever nature. The affair was equivalent to a picnic or a circus. Schools turned out so that the kids could help with the driving and so they wouldn't have to miss the fun. Families set forth early in the morning with calves in wagons, old women leading cows on ropes, kids driving, bulls fighting strange bulls. It was all very exciting and everyone had a good time. On one day we injected eleven hundred cattle belonging to one hundred and twenty-five owners, a job that would have required at least two weeks had I been obliged to visit individual farms. Most impressive to department heads was the fact that we could do an entire county in one week and costs dropped to around five cents per animal.

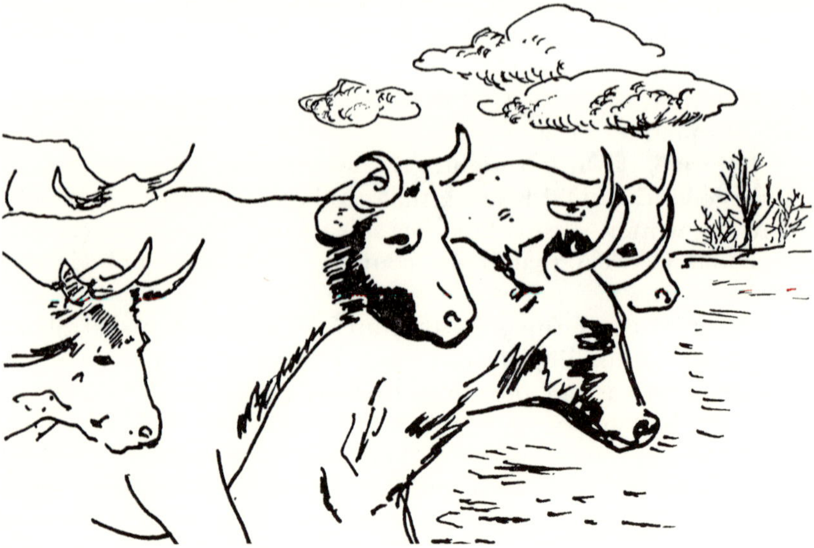

It goes without saying that in *any* disease control program *all* animals in an area have to be tested. None can be left out. "If you see any strays," we told the farmers, "bring *them* in, too." We were testing one morning when a young Indian boy came galloping in on a lathered horse, driving five yearling calves. "Strays," he told us. When we returned three days later for the reading, he came galloping in again with his five "strays," which passed with flying colors. We asked no questions.

With the Indians, language sometimes presented a problem. On the way to a reservation, once, I picked up a helper who lived in the area, hoping he could act as an interpreter. As we drove through the gate he said, "There's one thing. You'll have to do the talking, Doc. These people speak pidgin Osage."

"I don't know a *word* of Osage," I told him. "That's why I brought *you* along."

He stared at me in disbelief and disgust. "You mean you've gone all through *college* and still can't talk Indian?"

Coming into a strange territory, I always found it expedient to call first on the local sheriff, who would be familiar with the back roads and who might also know where I could find the farms I sought. Often enough, the sheriff would go along for the ride and this worked fine, too. If I ran into a recalcitrant owner who didn't want his cattle tested I found it handy to have the star and six shooter of authority aboard. This was rough country, with plenty of feuds still pending.

When I stopped one morning at the sheriff's office I found his uncle waiting. "Sheriff asked me to take his place," he explained. "He's laying low this morning and don't dare step outside."

"What's up?"

"The police chief is out to get him."

"What did the sheriff do to arouse the chief?"

"He shot and killed the chief's brother who was doing a little bootlegging. Got him with the goods. Shot the jug out of his hand and left a corpse holding the handle. The chief's pretty mad."

Occasionally we ran into a kind of puzzle. Each time I called in at one farm I found a few new reactors. The owner was getting rid of the branded animals all right and he couldn't figure it out either. One day when we were talking the matter over we fell to watching a little Jersey in the lot. She was chewing her cuds all right, but instead of swallowing them, then, she spat them out on the ground.

"She's been doing that for quite a while now," the owner told me. "I find cuds all over the cow lot."

"Let's just run her back into the chute," I told him. "I'd like to test her again." I knew there were rare cases so bad the animal failed to give a reading.

I gave her eleven shots of tuberculin an inch apart and went back in three days. She was a reactor and no mistake. The owner wanted her killed on the spot so that I could do a post and I finally consented, though I couldn't help wishing the children weren't around. It was obvious that she was an old family retainer. When the owner asked one of the boys to bring the cow, he jumped on her back and came lickety split, the way we used to do on the farm when we brought the milk cows in from the pasture. She looked to be in the pink of health.

Actually, I have never seen an animal so eaten up with tuberculosis. You couldn't have laid a quarter on her liver without setting the coin on a lesion. It was a great wonder the owner's family had escaped. I could only conclude that she was spreading the disease to the others by way of the spat-out cuds. He got the lot cleaned up and the reactors stopped.

Although the Texas fever control program had ended a number of years earlier, we still encountered farmers in eastern Oklahoma brush country who related and confused the two. They were always asking whether we intended to "dip" the cattle. Several of the older veterinarians we met had helped with the fever control and the stories they told were legion.

Unable to explain the importance of tick eradication to hill people who had grown up with ticks *(Boophilus annulatus),* they dipped everything they could find and were constantly on the lookout for strays. The disease lives inside the tick, an arthropod vector that acts as host. In order to facilitate the work, the tick country was laid out in fifty-mile bands, called "tick lines," that stretched all the way from the Mason-Dixon line to the Mexican border, in the hope of pushing the disease all the way out.

Workers tried to dip all the animals in a given area every nine days in order to wipe out ticks that remained in the brush and that would attach themselves to clean passing animals. When a cow emerged from the dipping vat her face was marked with paint. The men who did the rounding up and the dipping literally rode saddle. In pre-automobile days they took a train as close as possible to the tick area and then set out over the hills and through the brush on horseback. They did their own vat construction and hauled water in barrels on horse-drawn sleds over rough trails to fill them. Stories had gone the rounds to the effect that the dipping would kill the cattle, and many of the natives were up in arms. Occasionally workers arrived to find vats and barrels chopped to splinters.

One elderly veterinarian told a peculiar story about an owner who made a symbolic and senseless gesture of protest by arriving one morning with a rangy cow, plus a rifle held in the crook of his arm. Having announced, "You ain't agonna dip *my* cow," he raised the gun and shot the animal dead. One veterinarian was threatened so often with drowning in his own vat that he armed himself with a revolver.

Although the area was supposedly free of Texas fever before the tuberculosis program began, we, too, were always on the lookout for ticks. Of course there is no such thing as "eradication" of *any* disease; all we can hope for is reasonable control. As late as the 1930's veterinarians were still dipping in Louisiana bayou country. During the years when cattle were "trailed," that is, driven in herds across country, specific diseases moved along with the animals infecting the areas through which the animals passed. The Lord only knows how much Texas fever, or how much tuberculosis for that matter, moved over the famous Chisholm Trail. To be sure, when herds arrived in colder north country the climate eradicated the ticks. But a cow or two lost en route might well infect an entire area. With truck transportation and the present methods of strict inspection, the battle is a good deal easier.

When the tuberculosis testing program came to an end in Oklahoma, I received a request to transfer to Nebraska to work with the disease in hogs and chickens. B.A.I. researchers had worked out a theory that cattle were the source of infection in hogs and were trying hard to prove the validity of the belief, so it was a more or less pioneering venture. Bovine tuberculosis seemed pretty well under control, however, and the incidence on the hog packinghouse floor was not materially cut down. Our assignment in Nebraska was to help find the missing piece in the jigsaw. Our first station was at the town of Blair.

The new concentration on hog testing brought about a

revolutionary discovery. Hogs were found to be suffering not from the *bovine* (mammalian) strain but from the *avian* (poultry)! This revelation set us off on a new tactic. In those days the farmer's wife still raised most of the chickens, which were allowed the run of the hog lot. If avian tuberculosis were to be brought under control, perhaps the incidence of the disease in hogs would drop. It was an exciting challenge.

We began with a program of education, a slow process. My job, initially, was to follow up a letter mailed to each farm in a given township, to win the farmer's confidence, if possible, to explain the program, and to try to obtain permission to have a look at his flock. Occasionally through a process of deduction we were able to clear up an entire area. One case in point was that of a flock of fancy Nebraska Leghorns owned by a man I shall call "B." When we found considerable trouble among flocks owned by farmers who pointed with pride to the fact that their birds had come of B's Blue Ribbon stock, we made arrangements to visit B's hatchery. As with the Bar-X bulls mentioned earlier, we found that B's fancy Leghorns were spreading tuberculosis throughout the state.

I never really liked working with chickens, nor met a veterinarian who did. Partly, I suppose, this may have been a holdover from boyhood, when chickens were considered *woman's* work. This was pure snobbishness. But the fact that we felt pretty sure we were on track of something lent a new dignity to the research. When we had the disease pretty well cleaned up around Blair, I was asked to move up to West Point where there was a heavy incidence. Unable to find a suitable place to live, we settled on the nearby town of Wisner. Here, my continued work with tuberculosis was halted by the outbreak of World War II and a hitch in the Army Veterinary Corps.

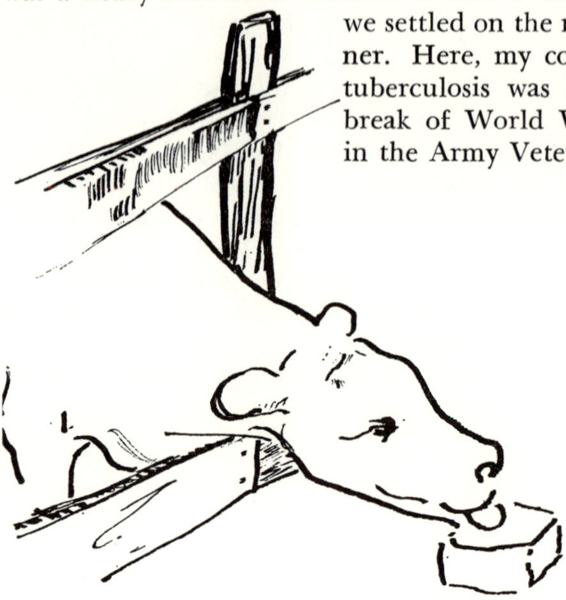

SOLDIERING

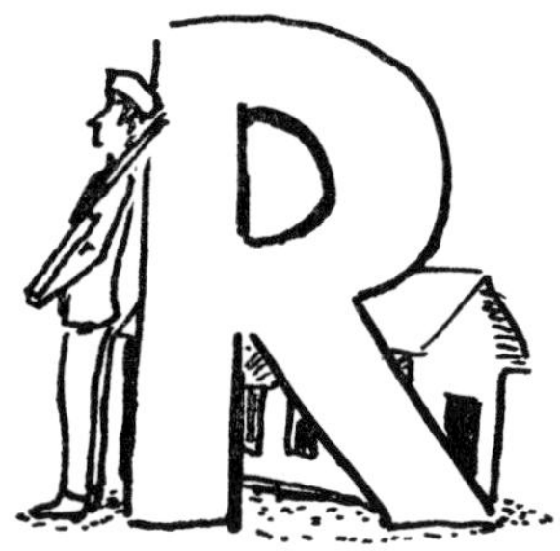

RESERVE OFFICERS' TRAINING, later to fall under a cloud because of the Viet Nam fiasco, had been a financial help during our college years. According to law, all male students in land grant colleges, such as Kansas State Agricultural (called "Cow College"), were obliged to undergo two years of reserve officers' training. Because of the stipend offered, many of us remained in the program for four years and continued in Reserves after graduation. One or two students in our small group entered the regular army as veterinarians.

During the first two years we had been required to drill along with other trainees from various departments, but for advanced R.O.T.C. we were placed in a group called the Veterinary Medical Corps, and only attended lectures. For this we were paid nine dollars a month, a not inconsiderable addition to the standard of living achieved by most of us. Upon graduation we were awarded the rank of Second Lieutenant.

As veterinarians, we were not called upon to undergo summer training. When money was available we did go somewhere for short refresher sessions. One of these, I recall, was held one year at Camp Travis in San Antonio. When I arose following a first night in an old World War I barracks, I discovered the sheet on my bed dotted with blood stains.

"Just bedbugs, old man," a veteran enlightened me. "You're not supposed to scratch." The entire barracks was crawling.

We also underwent brief periods of training at Camp Robinson, Arkansas, at Camp McCoy, Sparta, Wisconsin, and at Fort Robinson in Crawford, Nebraska. In 1934, by act of Congress, we were automatically promoted to the rank of First Lieutenant.

As potential Veterinary Corps men at school, we had been given much work in map reading, along with problems in traffic control. And, whereas I never really had any occasion to use this knowledge, I found the subject fascinating. One of our professors in R.O.T.C., a Dr. Fitzgerald, had served overseas during World War I, and often told of his experiences there. I especially recall one assignment he related. During a troop and equipment movement it was noted that shells were being thrown into a certain crossroads sector at definite intervals. By timing the speed of traffic and the rapidity of movement of certain of our sections to coincide with lulls between firing, he told us, the corps was able to take an entire contingent through without a single loss.

The average life of a horse on the front line, he said, was eight days, and large numbers of animals had to be destroyed. It was for this unhappy purpose that army veterinarians were finally allowed to carry sidearms. Disposal of dead animals at the front presented a problem, as such disposal had, ten times over, during the Civil War. It seems too bad that the deeds of these unsung animal heroes have been forgotten save by the old-timers who remain to tell about them.

During World War I, prior to our entry into the war, England had scoured the United States buying army type horses and mules to be used as cavalry mounts and as draft animals to move guns and supplies. This depletion resulted in our army experiencing considerable difficulty in obtaining horses for use after we entered the fray. I recall my brother Charlie, a member of an engineering train, having told of being issued *British* horses that responded, surprisingly, to the commands of "gee" (right) and "haw" (left). It is interesting to note that at one time during World War I, eighty percent of the United States army horses in Europe were incapacitated by mange and scabies.

Even during World War II, because of the shortage of gasoline, the Germans used some eight hundred thousand horses during their drive down through the low countries. On one occasion, a horse-drawn German army retreating east of Paris was surprised by an attack from a Canadian artillery unit that had hidden in the hills and zeroed in on the road the Germans were traveling.

Nearly all of the horses were casualties. A Texas sergeant in an American unit that came by, saw the remains of the debacle and shed tears, not over the dead soldiers but over the dead horses.

One problem we studied in R.O.T.C. and later in wartime training concerned the evacuation of animals in cases of emergency, such as bombing or gas attack, a responsibility to be assigned to the Veterinary Corps. Rules were essentially the same as rules for the evacuation of civilians.

When the war broke out in 1941 I was still working with tuberculosis. Indeed, the program went on all through the war, but on a retrenched scale because of a shortage of personnel. But I was on file in Washington, D.C. as having tested milk in Oklahoma, as well as on Army Reserve list; and so I was asked to transfer to the Public Health Department for inspection of dairy foods and other products at military bases.

Inasmuch as seventy-five percent of all foodstuffs are of animal origin, it made sense, I suppose, to require this work of members of the veterinary profession. Public health carried a number *two* priority, whereas animal industry made do with a number *five*. Had I declined to go, I would no doubt have been drafted. Following six weeks of training at Bethesda, Maryland, I was sent to the Kansas City regional office for six weeks' orientation and then assigned to the Pennington County Health Unit in the Black Hills of South Dakota.

Black Hills work alternated between Rapid City Air Base and Fort Meade Cavalry unit. One of my duties was to build up a sanitary milk supply in the area that "enjoyed" a sudden surge of population because of the influx of soldiers. I also inspected mess hall, milk, butter, ice cream, their sources, tested for butterfat, taught milk sanitation to nurses, checked water supply and sewage disposal, inspected restaurants frequented by soldiers, and worked with M.D.'s in an effort at control of venereal disease. On one occasion I was called upon, for some reason, to do a post exchange inventory.

According to regulations, I was to be accompanied on monthly inspection tours by two medical doctors; but this assignment was rarely carried out. Possibly the M.D.'s felt it a bit beneath their dignity to follow a horse doctor about, and I never blamed them. They had their own work, both time-consuming and strenuous, and there was a shortage of doctors. When a soldier fell violently ill one day and no M.D. was available, someone came for me. The soldier's wife, it developed, was in the habit of sending him packages of his favorite sausage halfway across the United States by surface mail, and he had partaken heartily of this viand. Miraculously, he survived. When I complained about being called in to look at a human patient, the M.D.'s were quick to point out that whereas human bellyache was, *indeed,* their responsibility, desiccated meat fell into the category of work for the Veterinary Corps.

On another such occasion, I flatly refused to function. I had been assigned, for some absurd reason, the title of "base surgeon" for two weeks. I suppose no one else was available. When a corporal appeared with a sick Navajo Indian in tow, I inquired what seemed to be wrong.

"If I were to take a guess I would say he may have appendicitis, Sir."

"Well, I'm not an M.D.," I said. "I'm a horse doctor. But tell him to lie down there on the table."

When I gave him a gentle jab in the side and he jumped two feet off the examining board that was all I needed to know. "Take him to Fremont," I told the corporal, "and get a medical doctor up there, *fast.*" I wasn't about to sign any death certificates.

Whenever we discovered a case of VD we made every effort to find the source before half the camp was infected. "But I never *asked* her name," one soldier insisted.

"Could you describe her for us?"

He said, near tears, "All I remember was she was a cross-eyed Indian."

Unable to find a single cross-eyed Indian girl within a wide area surrounding the camp, we were obliged to call it quits on that one.

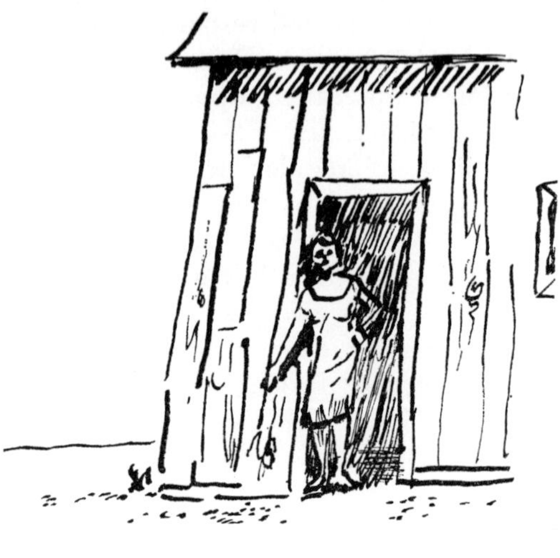

In January of 1943, after nine months in Rapid City, I was called back to active duty in the Army Veterinary Corps, which held an even higher priority than Public Health. From that time until the war ended, I was shifted from base to base. Water and milk supplies and general sanitation remained my immediate responsibility; but I was also called upon to perform a variety of duties ranging from service (for three months) as a judge on court martial cases to actual veterinary work with horses, mules, and guard dogs.

Contrary to popular belief that World War II was completely mechanized (as noted earlier), a great many mules and horses were pressed into service. Following "indoctrination" at Ponda, Colorado, and inspection, mules were shipped overseas for use on rugged terrain such as in Italy. Tough and intelligent, these animals did yeoman duty. While not so fast as a Jeep, a mule can go a good deal longer without refueling.

During the war, three remount stations were still active, at El Reno, Oklahoma, Front Royal, Virginia, and Fort Robinson, Nebraska. Horses used by the military were sent to one of these to be assigned. Along with certain other commodities, veterinarians, considered "lend-lease personnel," were in short supply for these bases. In line of duty, we sometimes collided with civilians out to make a fast buck off the army. I recall a set-to once with a theatre owner at Fairbury, Nebraska.

Having discovered a veritable scourge of bedbugs in the barracks, we suspected a probable source, a theatre that enjoyed a large soldier trade. Taking a few seats apart, we exposed literally thousands of these flat-bodied insects, and promptly placed the theatre "off limits." The owner screamed protest but hired an exterminator, who employed a "secret formula." Overriding the objections of the owner, who called to demand that we remove the off-limits sign, we took yet another seat apart. The joints swarmed with live bedbugs.

Among my unhappiest assignments were those as escort to the home-bound bodies of soldiers killed in non-combat here in the States. When two B-17s collided over South Dakota mountains, I was obliged to go to Sioux City, Iowa, to pick up a body to escort by train to Klamath Falls, Oregon. The dead soldiers had been brought out on horseback and reposed in forty-six caskets on the station platform.

An example of the way in which red tape can stretch to ridiculous lengths occurred at Scribner, Nebraska, where I served for a time as medical supply officer. Following reactivation of the base, a complaint came in to headquarters about the condition of the kitchen mess and I received an inspection order from the commanding officer.

The word "mess" was entirely appropriate. I made a long list of deficiencies. On the following day I was called in to the C.O.'s office to report. Having heard me out, the C.O. said, "That sounds terrible, Doctor. I'm appointing you mess officer. Go clean up that kitchen."

As mess officer (according to regulations) I was obliged to report to the medical inspector (myself) when I had finished an assignment. Kitchen cleaned, I wrote a letter to myself to the effect that as a result of a productive consultation with my commanding officer, I, mess officer, had cleaned up the kitchen as ordered, and sent a copy of the letter to the commanding officer. I suppose a copy of the letter from Dr. Price to Dr. Price may be on file somewhere among army archives.

One duty was to inspect canneries that put up K- and C-rations for army use. K-rations consisted of a highly concentrated food assembled and packed for the use of the isolated man who must be entirely self-sufficient, as in some forms of combat. C-rations were packed for the soldier farther back from the line. We naturally received a good deal of flak from individual soldiers about this type of food, but the rations were necessary and served the purpose for which they were intended. Our job was to see that specifications in the formula were met to the letter.

It was in connection with this work that I learned that an inspector's most valuable assistants are sometimes the employees on the assembly line. One day an indignant redhead assigned to the line came to me to complain about the beans being processed for the rations. "I've got a boy in the service," she told me. "I wouldn't want *him* eating this stuff."

The foreman tried to bluff. The only way *he* could correct the situation, he said, was to send some of the beans to the lab and get a directive. That got my dander up. I told him that no one in his right mind could look at those beans and judge them fit for human consumption. The simple fact was that no one was either looking or sorting. Maybe I couldn't condemn the lot, I said, but I could sure as hell stop the line until such time as he put on sufficient personnel to sort out the spoiled ones.

The army bought thousands of dollars worth of C-rations a day and a lot of plants were involved. Most of these did an honest job. The boxes were shipped, unsealed, to Kansas City, where a bread ration was added. Packages were made of some kind of waterproof material, so that in case of amphibious operations they could be dumped into the water and go in safely with the tide.

I am sure that "specs" in both food and clothing for military use have changed considerably over the years. It seemed to me that some changes were certainly in order. When orders came in for so many sides of "steer beef," we were obliged to comply literally with the directive. Once an animal is slaughtered and hung, it's pretty difficult to distinguish a steer from a heifer, and I would have to be shown that a soldier with a mess kit of steaming stew could tell the difference. But . . . confronted by specs and the carcass, we looked for the small opening called the "pizzle eye" through which the penis had emerged.

Equally wasteful of manpower and money, it occurred to me, was the fact that the army insisted upon writing its own milk regulations. The United States Department of Health had a fine standard milk ordinance, used by cities all over the country, that would have served as well.

One quaint regulation I frequently ran athwart of personally had to do with the complicated gobbledygook known as "travel pay." Travel pay is a bit of a joke in any case, being generally inadequate to cover expenses and based more or less on horse and buggy locomotion. In one instance my own travel allowance was cut to a cent per mile because the road over which I was obliged to pass paralleled a land grant railroad. Not taken into account was the fact that no train had been scheduled over the road for more years than anyone could remember.

A few veterinarians made it overseas but I was not one. For one thing, I was a bit overage. One younger vet I knew was assigned to the Gold Coast of Africa, where he flew back and forth over thousands of miles of desert terrain to inspect the egg and milk supply at an emergency air base.

In the spring of 1945, near the end of the war, I was stationed at Camp Ellis, Illinois, where a good many horses were kept. A number of old houses had been burned down in order to make room for the base. I suppose it would have been an all but endless task to pick up the nails and sift the ashes; but both humanely and economically the money would have been well spent, for the horses there suffered almost innumerable nail wounds in their feet.

In most cases, the injury was a simple prick, and at first we inserted a blunt needle and treated the small wound with iodine or some other dependable antiseptic. But then, approximately six months later, many of the horses turned lame and we found a pus pocket from a slowly developing organism. We learned to keep a record of which horses had picked up nails and the dates. If we had satisfied ourselves with the above treatment, we could almost peg the time when complications might arise. If we missed the initial prick, as we did sometimes, we knew, when sore feet and lameness occurred, that the animal had picked up one of the rusty nails in the area.

Ellis was an odd combination, a kind of project hodgepodge. Around thirty-five hundred prisoners, German, Austrian, Pole, and Czech, were stationed there; and the horses were kept for the guards' use, for work in the prison gardens, and for hauling trash. Too, shellshock cases returned to this country were sometimes brought to Ellis for rehabilitation, and some of these men rode horseback as therapy.

In addition, certain men were trained in survival at Ellis and sent out to work on the Alcan Highway, considered strategic at the time as some still believed that a Japanese invasion might come from that direction. When Ellis was cut from ninety thousand to around fifteen thousand men, leaving a number of buildings empty, someone conceived a notion that gas masks left over from the scare in the big cities could be stored there. Brought in by the thousands in carload lots, these unused commodities may be there yet for all I know.

A lot of good horseflesh was in the vicinity of Camp Ellis, a kind of center for showing horses owned by fanciers in the area. Elaborately appointed trailers fitted as tack rooms rolled into the show grounds and riders as well as horses were skilled in showmanship. As the vet on the base, I was sometimes called upon to act as "second starter" on the track during the races that were a part of the performances. When I saw the first starter's flag go down I put my flag down, and the race was on.

One day when horses and jockeys were lined up at the post awaiting the signals, one rider suddenly set out full steam, and, unaware that he was performing solo, rode hell-for-leather completely around the track, only to find that his adversaries had not left the post. To an angry query as to whether he had seen a flag go down, the jockey admitted defensively, but with considerable embarrassment, "No. But somebody yelled, 'Go!' and I went."

As the war drew toward a close, we had a good deal of work to do in phasing out, storing, and getting rid of army surplus and all that. The finest horse I ever owned, a stallion named Denmark Warrior, was more or less army surplus. He belonged to a colonel at Bruning, Nebraska, and I came by him through a lucky accident when that base closed in December 1944. The livestock judging book I had studied in college carried a picture of "Denny's" grandmother, Peggy Denmark, and I had admired the colonel's Warrior; but I certainly never thought to own him.

When orders came to phase out the base, the colonel asked me to get a railroad car to ship the horse to his home in Florida, for the use of his sixteen-year-old daughter. Of course the shortage of railroad cars was extreme then. The railroad people merely laughed at my request. Even a colonel couldn't get anything like a promise within months. In any case, I told the colonel, in all honesty and without connivance, that I didn't think a stallion of Denny's spirit was anything for a sixteen-year-old girl to ride.

The colonel must have taken me seriously, for presently the banker in charge of the financial residue at the base asked me what I would give for the colonel's horse. I knew I couldn't begin to pay what he was worth, and in truth I didn't know what I'd do with a horse if I had one, then. But to see Denny was to want to own him, and I said I reckoned I could pay two hundred and fifty dollars. He knew that I knew the horse was worth a good deal more than that.

"Well, if we have to *give* him away," he decided, "we might as well give him to *you,* I reckon."

I hauled Denny up to a farm I had bought on Union Creek and left him there with a tenant. When I got back to Camp Ellis in the spring of 1945 I ran across a sergeant who was going down toward Union, and asked him to bring the horse back to camp, thinking I might as well keep him around as long as I was there.

Denny entered his first show at Camp Ellis, ridden by an MP who had arranged for scattered friends to clap loudly whenever he appeared. The ruse influenced the judges not at all; the pair came in last in almost every category.

I was at Camp Ellis when the war ended. Ellis, too, had been phased out the previous year. But I had come back to care for the horses following a six weeks' stint at a Chicago meat and dairy inspection school, a popular assignment for members of the Veterinary Corps. I was discharged in January, with a Captain's commission, and my army career was over.

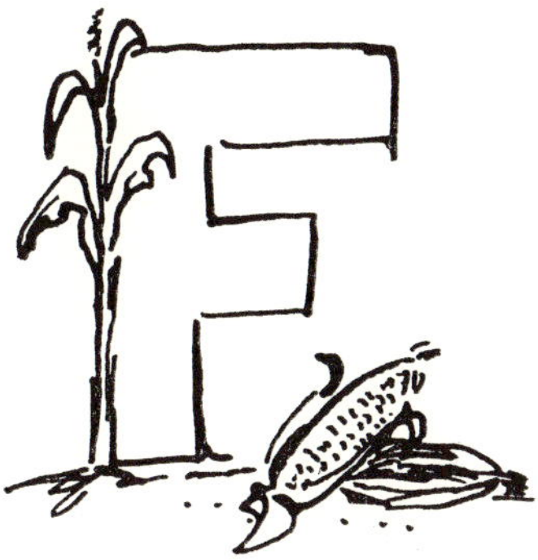

FOR SOME TIME prior to my return to Wisner, Nebraska, in 1946 I had been negotiating with Dr. D. O. Person, a retiring veterinarian, with a view to buying his practice. The tuberculosis program was being reactivated and stepped up, but I wanted to have another go at general practice.

We paid one thousand dollars for Dr. Person's practice, and set up an office in the basement of the public library. Supplies were difficult to come by, but we had a few left over. We acquired a Jeep and set to work. Three years later we built a combination home and office. We remained in Wisner until 1960 and wore out a total of nine Jeeps.

The northeastern Nebraska community differed about as widely as possible from Oklahoma Panhandle country. Corn and alfalfa largely made up the farm welfare, marketed through livestock. Farmers raised their own hogs but most of the cattle were shipped in as young stock and fed out. Many of these feeders were of German ancestry, with sons and daughters who had gone through agricultural college and come back with modern ideas.

Dr. Person, who had done considerable research on the subject, declared that more hogs were raised around Wisner than in any other twenty-five mile radius in the world. Agriculture there was a scientifically advanced industry, and Omaha had long since passed Chicago as a livestock market center. Signs reading THE BEEF CENTER OF NEBRASKA stood at en-

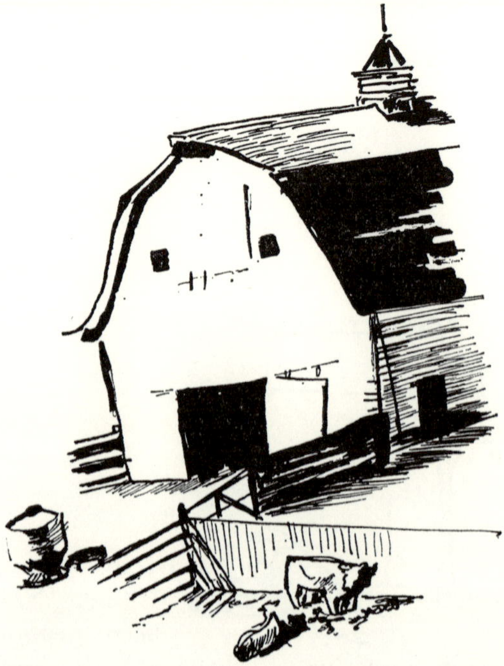

trances to the town of Wisner, and feeders met each morning at the elevator, as men meet on Wall Street, to view the "board" upon which the statistics concerning cattle and hogs moved through the previous day's "run" (market circuit) appeared.

Much of the feed used was mixed at the local elevator. Made up of corn, molasses, and various proteins, it went by the name of the "Wisner ration." Sometimes a drug, such as a hormone, was added. My own feeling concerning the use of such additives will be discussed in a later chapter. We came to especially appreciate one fact about these farmers, both large and small operators: they recognized that the treatment of an animal was a job for a professional. If a calf needed to be pulled or a cow suffered a prolapsed uterus, the owner called a veterinarian. Consequently, we encountered few of the half-finished or bungled jobs a vet comes to dread.

I hasten to say that we owed much of this ready acceptance to Dr. Person's well-deserved reputation. Educated in Canada, where veterinarians enjoyed a special kind of authority, he declined to allow his clients any more laxity than he accorded himself. A case in point occurred when he was called in once to attend a mare that had thrown her uterus. Having put the organ back in place, he instructed the owner sternly, "You're not to leave her for a minute, you understand. And don't sit at her head, but *behind* her. If she starts straining, get up and hit her with something soft, to distract her attention."

"My old man set behind that mare for three days," the farmer's wife told me," and held an old coat on his lap to larrup her with if she started straining. I had to carry his meals out to the barn and he only slept when *she* slept. He was that scared of Doc Person."

I never quite achieved *that* kind of authority, but I had no complaints.

One interesting and controversial condition we saw a great deal in the Wisner area, because of the movement, in and out, of feeder cattle was the pneumonia-like respiratory ailment we called "shipping fever." Both as a youngster on the farm and as a student, I heard much talk of "shipping fever," and I still read everything I can find on the subject. So far as I can learn to date, this disease (if it can be termed a disease) still baffles researchers, though it has become less frequent for a variety of reasons.

About the time of my senior year in veterinary medicine the state of Kansas appropriated some ten thousand dollars, a not inconsiderable sum in those days, to make a study of the condition. Because of differing points of view of two men involved, the study resulted in a bit of a fiasco and little in the way of resolution.

One theory concerned the stress and strain to which an animal is subjected during shipping. Another had to do with weaning; a calf, the same as a child, separated from its mother, undergoes a traumatic adjustment. And in many cases it was the newly weaned calves that were being shipped. About the time we thought we had come up with an answer, we hadn't. Tranquilizers added to feed were tried, in an effort to counteract the fever as well as weight loss incurred during the journey. But, administered wholesale, these took no account of individual weight differences; and overtranquilized animals were trampled to death by their fellow travelers. As a result of astronomical settlements, insurance companies finally declined to insure tranquilized cattle.

We did come to a few firm conclusions that seemed borne out by facts. We found that less time on the road resulted in less fever. A client who had bought animals in Montana had occasion to ship some by rail and some by truck. Both groups were loaded at the same time. When the trucks pulled in the following evening we found that group to be in good shape. The railroad car arrived four days later; and, for all that the animals had been unloaded and fed en route, their hair was dry, they were gaunt and dehydrated, and their eyes were filled with cinders.

Shipping in Nebraska followed about the same seasonal pattern. The first cattle came out of New Mexico and Arizona. Animals from Kansas followed, and then Wyoming and Dakota herds. Later in the fall they came from farther north and west. We came to note that the highest incidence of fever occurred in September and October, a fact that canceled the theory about cold wind in open stock cars. Indeed we noted time after time that the animals endured blizzard conditions far better than they tolerated heat.

Although we came no nearer to a knowledge of the real cause, the incidence of fever grew less as these abuses were avoided. Feeders bought bigger and older calves that had already gone through the weaning setback. Less shipping was done in hot weather. Good roads and faster and better-built trucks reduced time of exposure. And, as feeders bought directly from larger herds, the stockyards interlude that made for stress as well as possible contagion from a variety of herds from other areas was eliminated. Certain new immunizing agents came out and researchers began to suspect some viruses. We experimented with Terramycin and some of the sulfa drugs. We still saw death losses and setbacks that were about equal economically to death loss, but occasionally a bit of light filtered through and we were encouraged.

We still had with us, to be sure, the super-drug salesman from unethical companies, the brainwash ads that promised miracles to deluded stockmen . . . "eight hundred cases treated, with no death loss" . . . but we still had shipping fever. Asked the often recurring question at a state meeting, once, "What *causes* shipping fever?" pathologist Jack Ray came up with a classic answer.

"Shipping."

Whereas ours was not precisely scientific research, we felt we learned a good deal by simply exchanging notes on clinical experiences. One ailment we talked a good deal about was a condition in cattle we called "foot rot." We treated thousands of cattle for this, mainly with sulfa drugs after they were in better supply, and these proved effective. But we were constantly on the lookout for our ounce of prevention. The trouble was especially prevalent in the Missouri River bottom around Sioux City, Iowa; and so-called experts (of which there never seemed a lack) blamed unsanitary feedlots and frozen or rough, hard ground. But as far as we could discover neither condition existed in areas of the highest incidence. On the contrary, as with *erysipelas* in hogs, the disease appeared to *worsen* when animals were moved to dry, clean ground. These people were always suggesting we bandage the animals' feet. How we were to keep bandages on a cow running loose in a lot was not a part of the counsel.

Horses suffer from a different form of the disease, called "thrush," which affects the frog or sole of the foot; and with these, too, the condition appeared to be more prevalent in some sections of the country and the world than in others. We heard from a race horse veterinarian in Burma that veterinarians were encountering a very great deal of the trouble there.

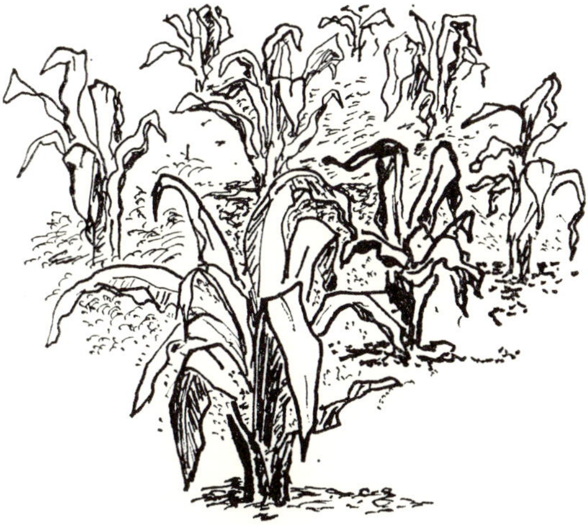

After I had been in practice in Wisner for a few years, I found myself up to my neck in community affairs. I served as mayor of the town for four years, as a member of the school board for eight years, and as a volunteer fireman in the all-volunteer fire department. We had some good fights but we also had a lot of fun. As mayor, I rode Denmark Warrior in many a parade, and he performed in a number of local shows. We often recall an incident when one of the boys who worked for us asked to ride Denny in a parade class, not realizing that the appearance of the rider counts for almost as much as does the aspect and behavior of his mount. On the day of the show Hazel and I sat in the stands, eagerly awaiting the appearance of the pair, and here they came. Denny shone from a thorough grooming and performed with his usual grace. In contrast to the other riders, in laces and colored silks, *our* boy appeared in ancient jeans and a battered ten-gallon hat, with boots and shirt that looked to have been resurrected from the city dump. Lest we be identified with the Warrior and his intrepid rider, Hazel insisted that we leave the show early and make our way out through the back.

Occasionally we allowed Denny to be used for breeding and he produced some fine saddle colts. But I always liked to be sure that his mates were worthy of his caliber. When a woman I knew only slightly called one day to ask whether Denny could breed her mares, I said, puzzled, "I didn't know you *had* saddle stock."

"Oh, I don't, Doctor," she told me airily. "But then I don't care anything about the colts. I just want to settle these crazy mares."

In 1952 we installed a two-way radio. Being able to contact home for calls that came in saved a lot of driving, as Hazel could send me from one client to another without my having to check in in person. She recalls a case I had forgotten. One day a client called in during a hail and windstorm such as we had occasionally, to say that his steers were bleeding badly from the jagged hailstones, as large as golf balls. When I drove into his yard, just minutes after he had called in, he would hardly believe that I had not simply stopped by for a visit.

Given good atmospheric conditions, the range of the two-way was remarkable; and we became acquainted with veterinarians as far away as Washington state. Once after Hazel had directed me to a calf-pulling job, she overheard a woman in Miami, Florida, tell a receiving friend, amid peals of laughter, that she had heard some woman tell some man to go somewhere and "pull a calf." Eighty percent of the calls that came into the fire department were country calls, and we found the two-way helpful there, too. To facilitate finding a fire, we had given each house a number, posted on a map at headquarters, where we kept two wagons and a tanker.

My fireladdy job was to prevent excessive damage and to render first aid when needed. One evening my son-in-law, Mike, and I, called to a car fire, went a little beyond first aid to unethically practice some human medicine. The fire occurred following an accident on a cold, windy night near the little town of Beemer and involved a drunk, a bus, and a pheasant hunter. Upon arrival, we found one man beyond help. The drunk, too far gone in inebriation to feel much pain, lay at the side of the road with a broken leg.

When Mike brought a big war surplus bandage and the hammer we used to kill hogs, from the Jeep, our friend roused enough to ask if we were doctors.

"Not medical doctors," I told him. "Veterinarians." The reply didn't seem to reassure him much, but he had little choice.

The hammer having failed to serve as we had hoped for splint material, Mike returned to the Jeep and brought the bolling gun, a metal rod with a cup at one end, used to administer medication to an animal in pill (bolus) form. No device could have worked better. Reasoning that our patient was too anesthetized to feel pain, we thrust one end of the gun into his shoe, pulled his leg into place, and set the bone.

When the alarm sounded on another cold night we rushed to headquarters, picked up the posted number, "906," and roared away with bells clanging. Finding a burning shed, we quickly extinguished the blaze. We were a bit longer placating the owner of the shed, who had carefully centered the structure over a frozen well and set it on fire in order to thaw the ice. By the time we arrived, red-faced, at "609," the chimney fire in the jeopardized house there had fortunately burned itself out.

A tricky, stubborn fire having broken out one Sunday morning inside the upper story of a house belonging to a character we called Jughandle Jones, we made the run full force and set dutifully to work, making every effort to confine the blaze to the single floor. Bursting through the back door during the height of the conflagration, I was outraged to find our host seated calmly at the kitchen table enjoying his morning pancakes. Pausing with a dripping morsel halfway to his mouth, he looked up to ask with interest, "How's it going, Doc?"

Occasionally our fire duties assumed the role of police work. One night around eleven o'clock a farmer phoned, in considerable distress, to say his wife had disappeared and that he could find no trace. The couple had been to town that afternoon, he related, and had returned home late, having stopped for a time at a tavern en route. Upon arrival, the husband had gone to milk the cows, his wife to gather eggs. He had not seen her since.

We searched every nook and cranny on that farm, without success. We fine-combed the woods, the ditches, the meadows, and the pastures on surrounding places. A few firemen gave up and went home. Increasingly alarmed, the rest of us stayed on, to fan out farther and to recheck, with flashlights, the area already searched. We were about to remarshall our forces at three A.M., when the missing woman walked in through the back door. She was furious. A great pity, she told us scathingly, that a woman couldn't go out for an evening stroll without the whole town getting into the act.

Although I knew, of course, that there was an element of danger, I had worked with undulant fever (brucellosis) a great deal, with no thought of personally contracting the disease. I can only believe that the fact that I did so while we lived in Wisner, following discharge from the army, resulted from my having worn out an earlier immunity built up through exposure. The ailment, as I entertained it, followed a symptomatic pattern. The name, which comes from "undulating fever," describes the happening. Each afternoon I ran a low grade temperature, that came on each day a little later. Many cases were fatal, but mine proved comparatively light. My doctor prescribed a sulfa drug, which put an end to the matter.

I like to remember that I had the pleasure of lunching, once, with bacteriologist Alice Evans, who proved that brucellosis in animals is contagious to the human system. Miss Evans' discovery was a genuine contribution in the field of research, as was that of Mr. B. L. F. Bang, the Danish biologist. Brucellosis is still known in some circles as "Bang's disease." To be sure, the bacterium *Brucella abortus* is only one of *several* organisms that cause undulant fever in man. Other names for the disease are "Malta fever," "Mediterranean fever," and "rock fever." A good many veterinarians (our son Dean among them) came down with the ailment during my time of practice. I suppose they still do. But thanks to a vigorous program of vaccinating and testing, brucellosis seems mercifully on its way into limbo.

I recall hearing a statement made around 1929 or 1930 by a Kansas state health officer concerning "Bang's disease," as he called it. "This might well be classed an industrial disease as it applies to humans," he declared, "inasmuch as most of the victims are either veterinarians or packing house workers who work with hogs." At that time, it might be noted, it was not yet known that the porcine variety was the most virulent of the strains.

It was while practicing in Wisner that we "enjoyed" an experience with an international exchange veterinarian. I hasten to say that ours was not typical of the exchange doctors. I expect that we in turn may have dispatched some bad ones to other countries. And at least he gave us a few laughs.

This particular exchange program had been set up between the University of Nebraska and the University of Ankhara, Turkey, in the hope that each could learn something from the other. The head of the program at Lincoln called to say that he wanted this particular doctor (whom I shall call Mehmet) to know something about the way we worked in the cattle-hog area. We were asked to take him in tow.

I'm not sure our visiting veterinarian learned much. Nor do I think he went home with a very high regard for either our work or our manner of living. Mehmet wasn't, he hastened to explain with no little pride, a full-time practicing veterinarian in his homeland. A combination Doctor of Veterinary Medicine and Medical Doctor, he held a chair of internal medicine at Ankhara. I don't really know what he hoped to learn by following us around; I came to think he had simply signed up for the ride. Close to his forties in age, he admitted to having been indulged by his "five grandmothers," that is, his grandfather's five wives. He didn't live with us, but he took most of his meals at our place. For religious reasons, he declined to eat pork, and we respected this. But if he himself were tempted by a dish that contained pork, he chose not to understand our explanation of the contents.

It being something of a novelty to have a foreigner in town, Mehmet was frequently entertained by the well-meaning townspeople. Whether grateful or not, he remained boorish and critical. He couldn't bear American coffee and he used three tea bags to make a cup of tea. Politically, he was anti-American, anti-English, and pro-German. He spent our Veteran's Day, November 11, regaling us with derisive remarks about this country's and our allies' part in the late war.

Besides subsistence pay of nine dollars per day, little of which he used for food or clothing (and none for soap), he received a fair salary. We had found him a place to stay with a woman who rented him a room at a low rate because she wished to be a good citizen. At the end of his stay she presented him with a modest bill. He declined to pay, and the bill was finally paid by the head of the program.

We were not above pulling his leg. During a 'coon hunt to which we treated him, a coyote tuned up in a nearby field and Mehmet asked in alarm what made the sound. "A coyote," we told him. "It's a kind of wolf."

Here was a fearful word he know. "How many are there? Shouldn't we hurry and get out of here?"

We tried in vain to explain that the animal was harmless and that one could sound like a dozen, but he feared an encirclement.

A Muslim, he was much interested in religions. I think he must have attended every church in the town. He approved of none of them. When we took him to dinner at our church, he ate with gusto the food served and then waxed bitterly and scathingly critical of a house of religion desecrated by the serving of food, a place of worship you entered without first removing your shoes. He was deathly afraid of all bulls. He not only declined to help to hold the hogs when we vaccinated; he disdained to even *watch* the operation. In Turkey, he informed us haughtily, a professional veterinarian never used his hands; his job was diagnosis. No one bothered to build chutes, he added, as there were always plenty of "underlings" to hold the animals.

"But these were the very things we wanted him to learn," the project head protested.

It occurs to me that it would have been interesting, if perhaps disheartening, to have heard Mehmet's report to his colleagues and students concerning the life and work of a veterinarian in the United States of America.

OPEN RANGE

My decision to go into brucellosis control and other work for the Animal Disease Eradication division of the United States Department of Agriculture in Nevada came about for a variety of reasons. We had built up a good practice in Wisner. Both our son Dean and our son-in-law Mike were graduate veterinarians. Mike had come in with me for a time and had done well. But the entire scene was changing and neither youngster really wanted to engage in private practice. The work had grown too heavy for me. I had picked up some rheumatism twinges and wanted to try a drier climate. And I was nearing an age for retirement.

Mainly, though, following a quarter of a century in Nebraska, I was hungry for range country again, and for open space. One factor that appealed to me especially about Nevada was its "bigness" . . . not the kind of bigness Texas boasts of, with Cadillacs and oil wells and money in wash tubs, but the spare wildness of open range and of semi-arid desert country.

As an instance, the area known as the Lazy-R (not the name) ranch where I spent two weeks inspecting cattle and writing health certificates for animals to be moved from Nevada to Montana comprised approximately four thousand square miles and included a United States bombing range. One reason I especially remember those two weeks has to do with two young girls encountered there.

After looking and driving about the West in search of a place, it occurred to me that I might have a fling at government work again, and here was an opening. I was given to understand that the work would be largely with brucellosis control but that there would also be some tuberculosis testing, with which I felt familiar, and some other chores such as the inspection of cattle to be shipped across state lines.

I never came to regret the decision to settle in Nevada. I have never worked with a people more hospitable nor more co-operative. Whenever we stopped at a ranch house we found a meal ready and an invitation to share it, American fried potatoes, wonderful homemade bread, delicious pies, (on one occasion) piñon nut gravy.

One ranch where we were especially well treated was run by a Mr. Pappiono. Shortly after leaving Nevada we read of Mr. Pappiono's death, and presently we received a note expressing appreciation of my having served as a pallbearer at his funeral, which I had not attended. We sent condolences to the Pappiono family and explained that there was some mistake for we had not in reality even known about the death.

We received a prompt reply. The family knew we no longer lived in the area. The note of appreciation had been sent, it was explained, because I would have been *asked* to serve had I still resided in the vicinity.

One problem we constantly encountered in Nevada was that of insufficient help for the roundup of animals to be tested. To use the Lazy-R again as an example: The grazing acreage spanned some one hundred and thirty-five miles in length by thirty-five to forty miles in breadth. To be sure, the land did not belong to the owner of the grazing herd; he owned only the portion upon which his headquarters were situated. The remainder was open range for which he paid grazing rights measured in "animal unit months."

In open range country where such use is made of public lands, animal unit months (known as AUM) is a term well understood, one AUM being the unit estimated to be necessary to sustain *one* cow for *one* month. A thousand AUM would, theoretically, support one thousand cattle for one month or one hundred cattle for ten months. For purposes of calculation, the AUM for five sheep would be the same as for one cow.

The owner of the Lazy-R herd (I will call him Roper) was

a bit of a gambler, as all big stockmen must be if they are to remain in business. Some said that he got his start with a "long rope and a fast horse," a phrase used for rustling; but I do not know that this was true. Some will always say this of a big rancher, and, big or not, Roper *thought* big.

When Roper decided to move his operation to Montana, we entered the picture as inspectors. Montana authorities required health certificates signed by a veterinarian who had made a clinical observation. To range over four thousand square miles of mountainous country rounding up cattle is no small task, and so we did the job piecemeal. The new ranchers had brought in cattle of their own, with their own brand, and there developed some controversy between them and Roper concerning newly dropped calves. Roper had asked for a year in which to get his cattle off the range and the newcomers accused him of dawdling, claiming that the supply of grass was being depleted by his tardiness.

Meanwhile, we heard indirectly that Roper had run into difficulties in Montana because of the delay, having persuaded certain Montana bankers to finance his new setup by agreeing to place a given number of animals on the new range by a set date. The first load of animals had arrived; but then the state authorities had declined to accept the signature of a "fee inspector" of brands without that of a veterinarian to back it up.

Hazel and I were on a combination business and pleasure trip to Lake Tahoe when I received a call asking me to examine the animals and to write certificates of health inspection. The cattle were not yet rounded up, and the small corrals to which they were to be taken for examination lay some twenty to thirty miles apart.

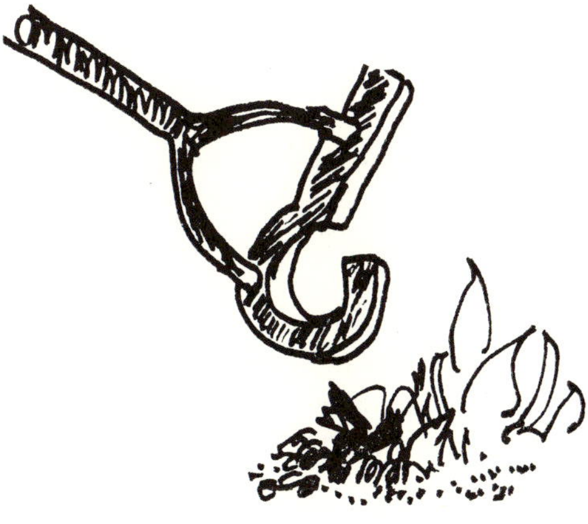

According to the somewhat hodgepodge plan, the driver who was to truck each given group of animals to Montana had been requested to call and inform us where these corrals were located.

Having received such a call, I set out with the brands inspector under such directions as "ten miles north of the old stone cabin" (a tumbledown structure once occupied by a settler in the area), or "ten miles east . . . or north . . . or south." We might well arrive and find an empty corral, necessitating a drive to a second or a third, which might or might not be tenanted.

If we found a herd waiting, Shirley Robinson (the brands inspector) checked to be sure the animals bore Roper's brand. My job was clinical. The trouble I found was largely "cancer eye," a condition affecting many whitefaces in that country. Frequently we started at two or three o'clock in the morning. Eventually we might find a corral partially filled with wild-looking animals and the trucker waiting, or *he* found *us* waiting. The trucks were two-storied affairs described as "possum-bellied."

It was at one of these corrals that we first encountered the Roper girls. Around fourteen and sixteen years of age, they were every bit as tough as the animals they lived with. In the saddle all day, these kids slept wherever they chanced to be when night fell, wrapped in dirty blankets, in the truck that carried the horses the fifty or seventy-five miles to where they were needed, in some abandoned shack on the range. The roundup of one small herd ended at a neighboring ranch one night around nine.

"Seeing how haggard and beaten the kids looked," the ranch wife related, "I asked when they had eaten last. One of the girls recalled they had had breakfast around six in the morning. I set to work to fix a meal. The girls leaned against the wall for a while and watched, and then slid to a sitting position. The next time I looked they had fallen over, dead to the world."

Having received word one morning that a number of animals had been corraled close to the bombing range, we set out earlier than usual, and drove for hours over miles of rugged terrain without any sign of civilization. Around noon we were flagged down by a foreman employed by the incoming ranchers, who advised us to leave our car and ride along in his truck. "It gets rough out there," he told us. "You couldn't go much farther in that rig."

We found the corral at approximately four o'clock in the afternoon, a beaten up loading chute that bristled with splinters and fifteen head of wild cattle. One of the new ranchers had engaged in fisticuffs with Roper over a calf he claimed Roper had branded. Having ridden up and down many canyons in order to round up the few animals, the Roper girls sat quietly on their mounts, awaiting further orders.

"The canyons were filled with wild horses," the youngest told me. "Some of them looked awful."

I would like to say a word here about these pathetically inbred horses, many of which were cruelly deformed. A stallion would round up a band of mares and take them into the canyons, keeping them there for years and breeding his own daughters and granddaughters.

I have seen a good many untamed cattle in my time, but these fifteen animals the Roper girls had rounded up took the oatmeal cluster for sheer wildness. We handled calves four months old that had never laid eyes on a human, calves to which man in whatever guise was ENEMY. They put their heads down and charged anyone who entered the corral. When I tried to examine them they fought like wildcats. I didn't wonder that the girls looked exhausted. I asked whether they had had anything to eat. "We ate this morning," the youngest told me.

What time had they left camp?

"I reckon it was about six," she said.

I had emergency food in the car. But it was back ten miles or so. Having heard our conversation, Roper went to his car and came back with a can of pears and one of tomatoes. He opened the cans with the long blade of his jackknife, stabbed pear and tomato and fed them to the girls in turn, as they opened their mouths like fledglings to take the morsels from the knife point.

As we sat waiting for the truck to load, I asked the girls whether they attended school during the winter months.

"Sometimes we go," one told me.

People were wont to say that Shirley Robinson had eyes like an eagle. Frequently as we drove along he would make a count of deer on some mountainside where I could see nothing at all. One morning as we were driving across range in search of some elusive corral he pointed out a little puff of dust some three or four miles across the desert.

"There comes one of those Roper kids," he told me, "driving a cow and calf."

The temperature stood at one hundred degrees in the shade, if you could find any shade. Training the glasses on the wisp of dust, I made out the youngest Roper girl perched on her big buckskin in the wake of a cow and calf. She seemed to be in some kind of trouble. The cow would break at a dead run and whirl back toward the hills and the girl would wheel and ride hell-for-leather in pursuit. We stopped to wait.

As the foursome approached we could see that both horse and cow were lathered. The girl looked simply beat. She asked whether we had any water and I got out my jug and asked her whether she had eaten. I had nothing in the car that day, but Shirley had a box of cookies. As she sat resting and munching, the cow broke suddenly and took off across the range. The girl spurred her horse and was off. As we watched the chase I remarked to Shirley that I never expected to see tougher cows, tougher horses, nor tougher kids, and I never have.

A few days later I asked one of the truckers if he thought the girls would be insulted if I gave them some food to carry along.

"Hell, no," he said. "Those kids will eat *anything,* no matter where it comes from."

I rummaged through my car and came up with a can of pineapple, some pork and beans, Vienna sausages, and a box of crackers. I even added a pan, in case they had an opportunity to heat the beans over a camp fire. On the following Sunday I met Roper and the girls about forty miles farther north. The girls handed me the can opener, the spoons, and the pan, and gave me polite thanks. Neither had previously tasted pineapple. Both thought it "wonderful."

The roundup was almost over and I told Roper I was leaving for New York on Monday morning to attend the American Veterinary Medical Association meeting. Roper replied that he guessed he was leaving, too; it was time to go on to Montana and start branding calves. That was the last time I saw any of them. I heard later that the girls had married, and wondered whether they had it any easier as ranch wives than they had as cowhands. I suppose either of them might well have teamed up with most any kind of cowpoke in order to get away from the kind of life she led.

Whether or not Roper was any kind of rustler, the country did harbor a few of the breed. Mostly they were small-time operators, out for meat. Catching a calf on the range, they would slaughter the animal on the spot, take the meat and leave the remains. With one pair from McGill, rustling proved something less than the perfect crime. Driving away from the scene, through

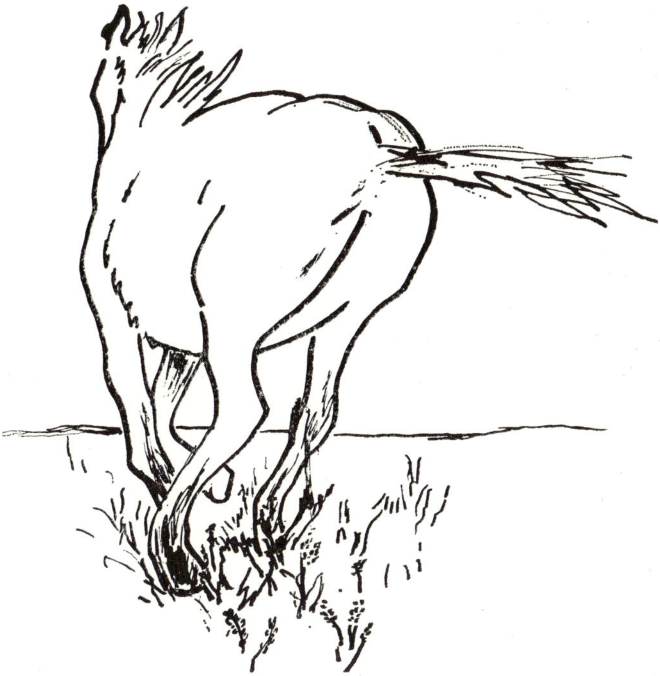

heavy brush, they lost the license plate off their car, which was picked up by the sheriff.

Having been dispatched to the town of Glendale one hot summer day to test a herd of Brahmas, some of which belonged to the local sheriff, I became aware as the day grew hotter of a purely-awful, stomach-filling aroma. Looking about, I discovered the source, an over-ripe cow's head lying in the nearby grass, and asked for its removal.

"Sorry," the sheriff told me. "That's evidence."

The little foreman told me the story, and made a wry face. The owners of the cattle, including the sheriff, he said, were investigating the loss of some missing animals when they noted flies buzzing about an old mine shaft.

"The shaft was around forty to fifty deep," he related, "and we couldn't see the bottom. Somebody found an old bucket and tied a rope on it and I was elected to go down, being the only one small enough to stand in the bucket. I found the attraction all right. Rustlers had killed a calf and dumped the offal and the hide with the brand on into the mine shaft and the flies had found it. Figuring the thieves might still be in the neighborhood, hanging around the trailer houses down by the road, the whole gang took off to make a search and left me down there with all them guts and stuff. I yelled my head off but it was close onto an hour before anybody remembered to come back and haul me out."

At the very first trailer house, he went on to say, the sheriff had found fresh meat after showing his badge and demanding to see the contents of the refrigerator. Every trailer owner in the camp had shared in the spoils.

Most ranch foremen, who drove about in trucks, carried rifles, in case they came across marauding coyotes or mountain lions after the calves. When one of these came abreast of a strange pick-up one day with a familiar-looking calf in the back he tried to hail the driver. But the fellow just stepped on the gas. The foreman shot two tires flat and punctured the gas tank, and then held the driver at gunpoint until the next car came along. He asked the occupants to notify the sheriff.

Actually, this area was pretty poor range country, the kind of semi-arid land that seemed to bear out the adage that man had, indeed, gone too far west with the cow. "The only kind of vegetation that survives the weather and the overstocking of herbivorous animals," one rancher remarked, "is either too thorny to eat (cactus, wild rose, greasewood), too woody for forage (rabbit brush and sage), or downright lethal."

Because of poor sustenance, ranchers could count on only about a thirty percent calf crop. A heifer might raise her *first* calf all right, but then be so suckled down that she would fail to breed back for two or three years. Gunnysack Robinson's "missmeal cramps" was a disease as comon in Nevada as on the Oklahoma range. As a government employee once more, I was not supposed to engage in private practice. But, as in Oklahoma, the nearest veterinarian was some ninety miles distant and I was often called upon, especially in an emergency.

One night around midnight I had a distressed call from a farmer whose burro had collided with an automobile. In open range country, with no herd laws, an animal more or less has official right-of-way, but that hadn't helped any. The little donkey was a mess, with a tooth knocked loose and a nasty cut that ran through his lip and down through his jaw. I found him standing patiently in a pool of blood surrounded by silent and grieving adults and wailing children, a beloved member of the farmer's family.

The sobbing and the screaming continued as I gave the burro

a shot of nembutal, waited for him to fall asleep, and set to work at the patch-up, removing the tooth and stitching up the cuts and abrasions. I could only hope he would survive, and obviously he did just that. For, years later, after we had left Nevada for the Pacific Northwest we saw an advertisement in the Nevada paper to which we still subscribed stating that the family's beloved burro was lost and pleading for his return. With that scar, it occurred to me, he would be easy enough to identify.

On most of the ranches, as had been the case during the drouth in the Panhandle of Oklahoma, the lack of water was a major problem. Mountain-fed creeks dried away in summer. For months at a time water was hauled long distances for livestock and domestic use, over roads that were little more than trails, faint and difficult to follow. Frequently I arrived at a ranch for testing only to discover that the last and longest leg of my journey was to be on horseback, or that I was expected to help with the roundup. A case in point was the Reese River Indian Reservation, where I found a diminutive, bowlegged woman waiting with a horse for me to saddle and ride. I have ridden many kinds of mounts in my time, but for utter lack of spring in motion this one took the prize. He moved as though all four legs were made of wood, a carved, unjointed part of the rest of his anatomy. When we had the cattle underway I began to notice that one cow was breathing uncommonly hard, and reined up just as she dropped dead, of emphysema. I could only protest to my fellow rider that he had only to take a close look at my noble steed to see that I had at least not *run* her to death.

It was during my sojourn in central Nevada that I underwent a peculiar transformation that remains to this day a mystery without satisfactory explanation. I lit up!

One night in our home in McGill, Hazel awoke and then woke me in alarm to point to the fact that I was glowing like a glowworm or a flying firefly. When I drew my hand across the sheet the fingers left five glowing trails in a ghostly pattern. Because of our proximity to the test area, we thought at once that I had somehow become radioactive, and called the Civil Defense authorities in the town of Ely.

A pair of reserve officers in town on special assignment for the Atomic Energy Commission went over me with Geiger counters, tested the bed, my clothing, my car, and found nothing. I was given a gadget to wear in my pocket, designed to detect radioactivity, but it, too, failed to produce results. I slept outside in the camper, parked in the back yard, and glowed as brightly as in my own bedroom. I felt fine and went about my work as usual. During the day I was completely normal. When darkness fell, I turned on. People who heard of my incandescence looked unbelieving. Or they laughed uproariously and without compassion. "If Doc turns on tonight," one called to say, "invite me over." I could have charged admission.

A visiting physicist from Northwestern University, sent to see me, came to a conclusion. The phenomenon resulted from "a combination of nylon with the detergent used [by Hazel] in the washing machine." But half the town used the same detergent, and I *wore* no nylon.

The odd business continued for a month or more, and then my moment as a shining star was over. The nearest anything-like-acceptable explanation had to do with the fact that I had been working prior to the first discovery on an alkaline flat, where I may have somehow become exposed to a combination of chemicals that resulted in a kind of phosphorescence. As did the Unidentified Flying Objects, I attracted rather wide local attention for a time, and became the butt of innumerable jokes. Then I flickered out. But I still receive an occasional letter from Nevada reminding me of my one brilliant episode.

Although our work in Nevada continued to be largely with brucellosis control, I was called upon now and then to test for tuberculosis. One test proved an interesting and rather precarious experience. The herd to be tested, consisting of some fifteen hundred Holsteins and Guernseys in a big dairy, was known locally as "the million dollar show herd." The situation as I found it was not to my liking. Arriving on the heels of another government inspector, I found thirty-three cows already tagged as suspects (from a previous test), the entire herd under quarantine, and the owner extremely disturbed. To add to the confusion, six other animals previously tested and condemned had gone to the packing house, where the meat had shown no signs of tuberculosis lesions. As second veterinarian in the field, I landed squarely in the middle of the controversy.

Because of the size and reputation of the herd, a number of people were interested in the outcome. I arrived to find a not altogether happy audience on hand, including the man in charge of tuberculosis control for the area and six or seven other veterinarians.

Twenty-one of the thirty-three tagged animals showed *no* reaction, the remainder only a trace. Ten or fifteen others out of the herd of seven hundred and fifty tested (that had not previously reacted) showed a trace reaction. We were puzzled and the owner was distracted. Entering a stall where I was at work, he asked if I had any notion of the value of the cow under examination. "I could get ten thousand dollars for her," he declared, "from any one of several sources."

As currently testing veterinarian, the decision to condemn or not to condemn was ostensibly up to me. Having carefully studied the reactions, I expressed the honest opinion that there was no tuberculosis in the herd. I was bound to admit some small reactions, I told the group, but I was sure they came from some other protein sensitization. The fact that twenty-one head of the thirty-three condemned had already cleared, I argued, pointed to a *transitory* condition, and there is nothing transitory about tuberculosis. I realized that I might get my head chopped off, but I was sure I was right.

Questioned closely, the owner admitted that two of the three classed as reactors had received several days' treatment with penicillin for unrelated foot ailments. Genuinely skeptical, and also on the defensive, the government inspector insisted that the three with the strongest reaction be sent to the slaughterhouse. They, too, showed no lesions. The entire herd was re-tested, without my help, this time with *no* reactors.

Because of the long quarantine period, the rancher was all but ruined. Disheartened by the setback, he sold out. To me, this was outstanding and painful proof that such a test, however valuable, is only a diagnostic aid. We have a tendency sometimes to place too much quick reliance on laboratory research as end and answer. Pressed for a definitive answer to some clinical question, Dr. Reed, a bacteriologist with the Norden Laboratories, used always to counter with the summation, "Of course there is nothing *sure* in biology, except death."

I had more than one reason to remember that particular event. Crowded against a fence during the testing, I suffered a broken rib, an injury quite as painful when inflicted by a ten thousand dollar cow as by one priced at twenty.

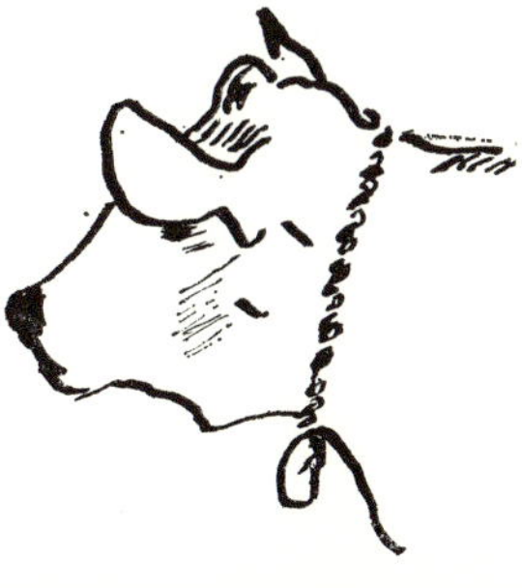

BASQUE

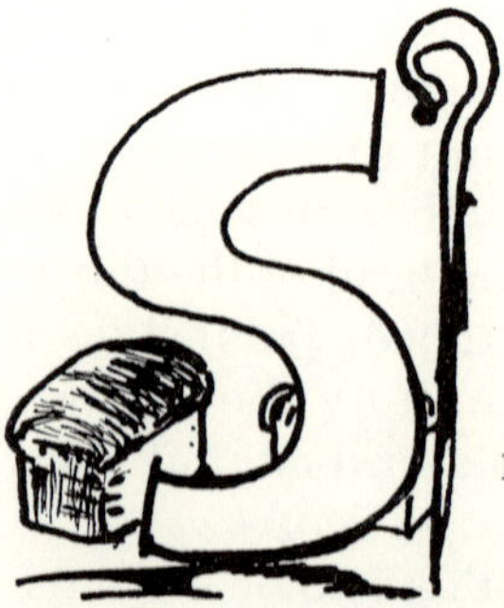

SHEEPHERDERS in the open range country of Nevada were largely of Basque origin. Living a solitary existence with their working dogs, they mostly held contracts for three years' work. Many returned, then, to their homeland; but some remained to take out citizenship and not a few became ranch owners on their own. Even of those who returned, many re-applied and came back.

Basques had been coming into the area from the Pyrenees mountain land shared by France and Spain for nearly one hundred years. It was estimated that these and their descendants scattered about over Nevada, Idaho, northeast Oregon, western Colorado, southwest Wyoming, central Arizona, and the Sierra Nevada Mountains of California numbered more than fifty thousand. We knew ranchers who bid high for the services of certain individual Basques who had proved their worth. Even on a cattle ranch, Basques kept a few sheep, and we were sometimes called upon by a flock owner.

Although we had treated sheep in both Oklahoma and Nebraska, we had never had much occasion to work with these animals. But we did what we could. The old saying that "a sick sheep is a dead sheep" is not necessarily true. I reckon the saying may have come from the fact that a single sheep is not worth very much and because you come to think of these animals in terms of flocks rather than as individuals. Too, sheep seldom display readily diagnosed symptoms, as most other animals do, and their diseases are peculiar to the species.

We occasionally saw a condition in Nevada known as "over-eating disease" (enterotoxemia) which recalled a sad experience we had in Nebraska. A client had purchased a preventive entero-toxemia vaccine from a drug store and had vaccinated six hundred feeder lambs a week previous. The lambs were sick and he was losing them quite rapidly, one hundred and fifty having already succumbed. I called on Dr. Ben Griffith, who was then working for the state of Nebraska. He took specimens to the laboratory in Lincoln, where it was determined that the lambs were dying from tetanus (lockjaw). Furthermore, live tetanus organisms were discovered to be present in the vaccine.

I suggested to the client that he contact the house that had sold him the vaccine and ask them to send a man out. I have rarely met a surlier or more belligerent character. He was, of course, on the defensive, and I guess our trust of each other was about mutual.

Another interesting if baffling disease we encountered in Nevada Basque country was known locally as "the stiff lamb disease," an ailment obviously associated with a mineral lack. When the university laboratory asked us to take blood samples to see whether they could get to the bottom of the trouble, we drove out to a ranch where only Basque was spoken. One reason I especially remember this experience has to do with the finest Border Collie I have ever seen. That dog had no need of *any* language. The herder motioned silently; the dog watched the gesture and responded with instant obedience. Just watching the pair at work more than compensated for the long drive.

The annual Basque festivals were lively occasions, with dancing and woodchopping contests and much good food and drink. The principal dishes consisted of mutton and chick peas, called "garbanzos." Men carried goatskin flasks known as "botas" from which wine was squirted into the bearer's mouth. A special drink called "picon," sweet and bitter, was served in filling station bars. Wine was made in cement vats from grapes shipped in from California. The beverage was drawn off at the bottom of the vat, from underneath crushed stems, seeds and skins, and was very sour. When one shipment of sheep left for a California market, the Basque escort took along one hundred and twenty-three gallons of the beverage for consumption en route.

Sourdough bread, baked in Dutch ovens, was indescribably delicious. At Basque tables you were handed the entire loaf, along with a knife, to serve yourself. The first meal of the day consisted of coffee poured over slices of this bread and served in bowls along with cream and sugar. Breakfast at midmorning might be a hearty omelet filled with bacon and potatoes, along with red beans seasoned heavily with garlic or mutton and onion stew. Dessert consisted of jam or canned peaches served in tall stemmed bowls.

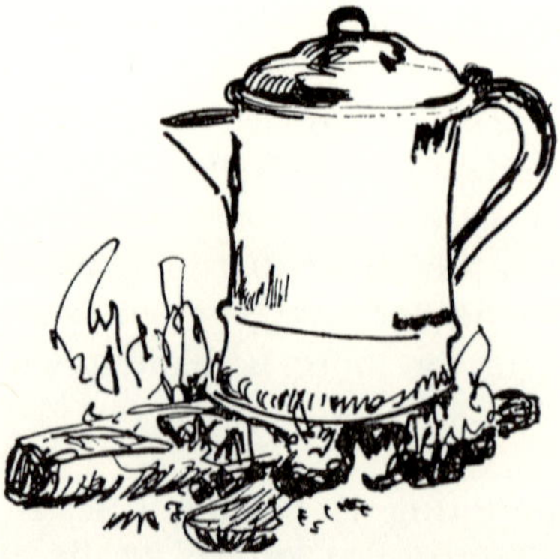

Sometimes we experienced a bit of difficulty with the language, which was neither French nor Spanish, but "Basque," a tongue that seems as shrouded in mystery as is the origin of the people themselves. Some say the Basques came originally from the Holy Land and that they have succeeded in remaining a remarkably pure strain. Of medium to small stature, they were almost without exception athletic, tough, clannish, and very clean. When we tested a herd, one day, confined to a too-small turnout pen, the Basque hands put on quite a show. They would poke the animals between the rails, dodge behind the scale and pop up and down like jumping jacks to get out of the way of the charge. The badly scarred face of one, it was explained, had come of his having bitten off a dynamite cap.

During our travels about the ranges, we often saw herders with their bands of sheep (consisting of around two thousand animals). These men lived a nomad and lonely life, moving from south to north as the seasons changed and back again over sagebrush country and juniper-clad hills, with only their dogs for company. During the drive, the animals were allotted a one or two mile strip for grazing, depending upon the number of sheep in the flock. Waterholes were few and far between. *White* sage was considered a choice food. Animals that ranged beyond their limit were brought back by the herder's dog.

A single herder, with his flock, might well drift as much as three hundred miles in a year's time. These men, in Stetson hats, boots, and with long staves, came to be a familiar sight on the solitary desert where they passed their lives. The trailer-like camp wagon was sometimes pulled by a pickup truck, but more often was drawn by horses that had outlived their usefulness for riding and roping. Furnished with a bed, a bench, and a small stove, these small dwellings on wheels were kept immaculately clean.

To protect the flock from coyotes and mountain lions, and to help with the drive, the herder might have one, two, or as many as five dogs. Largely black and white in color, these admirable animals were carefully raised and trained, the breed kept as pure as was possible. Two or three times a week, a check might be made on the herder from headquarters, but otherwise he was alone and responsible for his flock.

But, for all the solitude of their working lives, these were a gregarious and fun-loving people. Having gone into Basque country once to vaccinate calves, I drove from ranch to ranch without finding anyone at home. Learning, finally, that a Basque had died, I made my way to his house to express my regrets. The funeral had just ended and the mourners were departing in a group. "Come on along down to the saloon, Doc," they invited. "That's where we always go after a funeral."

I entered the saloon, to find the entire party on hand and really whooping it up. Having returned a year or so later to one of the ranches for some work, I said by way of introduction, "I'm Dr. Price from McGill."

"Oh, I remember you, Doc," came the prompt response. "You bought me a drink at K's funeral."

One Basque for whom I did some work, a diminutive fellow with a squeaky voice, lived west of Persimmon Flats. Having invited me into his house when the work was finished, he hopped nimbly onto a table and asked me to give him a boost through a kind of trapdoor in the ceiling. He reappeared presently with my fee, in silver dollars. A rancher to whom I related the incident interrupted my story, "Oh, I know who that was. That had to be Squeaky Beard. Everybody knows that's his First National Bank up there."

Many of the ranchers, though, were pretty hard up. I recall a visit Hazel and I made once to a shack sided with corrugated iron, set squarely in the middle of the desert surrounded by magnificent mountains. When Hazel remarked to the ranch wife about the loveliness of the view on all sides, a surprised look came over the woman's face. "I never have time to look," she said truthfully. After her husband died, she lived on at the ranch with her son, still working from daylight to dark, still unaware, I reckon, of the matchless beauty around her.

East central Nevada was good hunting country with plenty of meat game such as deer, sage hens, and waterfowl; and I sometimes took time out to do a bit of hunting with some of the ranchers. I recall especially one companion who stoutly insisted that he could distinguish a buck deer from a doe in the darkness by the color of the animal's eyes. "A buck's eyes are *blue,*" he asserted. "There's just no chance of mistaking him for a doe." He may have been right, too. Suiting action to his word, he blasted away one night at a blue-eyed target. The lantern revealed, alas too late, a Jersey cow.

We still laugh about a rancher named Herbie. When Herbie's mother died I called to express regret and said, "If there's anything I can do for you, Herbie, just give me a call." He said, "I'll do that, Doc." And he did. After several weeks had elapsed, I was awakened one night from a sound sleep by the ringing of the telephone.

"This is Herbie, Doc. Remember, you said to call if there was anything you could do for me? Well, I've got shingles here for a new barn roof and need help to nail them down tomorrow. And stop and bring Jack with you if you don't mind. I'll need all the help I can come by."

BRUCELLOSIS

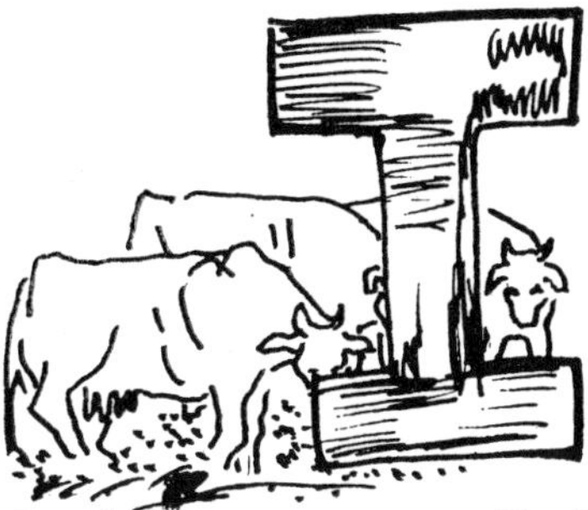

I REALLY CAME IN on the shank end of the brucellosis program in Nevada, most of the area having been already put on an accredited basis so far as this disease was concerned. But if an area is to *remain* accredited, herds must be tested every three years.

The only case of brucellosis we knew about on the home farm back in Kansas occurred in a neighbor's herd and all but whipped him out of business. Then, and there, the disease was known as "contagious abortion," and naturally all the stockraisers in the area were apprehensive. Someone contacted the county extension agent and he agreed to come to the rural schoolhouse and talk on the subject. A considerable crowd gathered.

As I recall, his remarks were anything but comforting. He told us there was no cure for the disease. One thing he did, probably, was to keep the farmers from loading up on quack, sure-fire drugs such as Bowman's Abortion Cure, a much-publicized concoction of bran and brown sugar that continued to be sold in appalling quantities for years afterward. However, I am bound to admit that the dissemination of this highly touted mixture was no more unethical than is the distribution of hundreds of patent human medicines advertised on the television screens to this day.

Largely our testing in Nevada was done on a percentage basis. If we ran into reactors we tested the entire herd, of course.

And we did a lot of vaccinating. When we found a seemingly definite reactor, we put a hot iron B brand on the left jaw and a red "condemned" tag in the animal's ear, and filled out papers for a government inspected slaughter house. A cow infected with brucellosis, I hasten to say, shows no lesions, as does one infected with tuberculosis, and the meat is entirely fit for food. To be sure, the carcass may be condemned for other reasons. Sometimes we made use of "back tags" for marking, a practice, incidentally, that was responsible for the development of the best doggoned glue ever invented. A lot of research had gone into the making of a waterproof paper that would hold up on a cow's back in all kinds of weather and a glue that would hold the tag to the animal's hide. The end product of that research held so tenaciously that it came to be referred to as "vet's baling wire," and "backtag glue" became a byword, not only for any *mending* job, but, figuratively, for anything that might otherwise become unstuck.

In the winter and spring we vaccinated heifer range calves. The job was not without its hazards. Every now and again we heard of some veterinarian who had jabbed himself with a needle by accident and fallen sick with undulant fever. A few died of the disease. A live vaccine is nothing to fool with.

The fact that some swivel chair doctor of veterinary medicine back in Washington, D.C., could order a given length of needle for these injections sometimes gave me a slow burn. Our objections (or more probably our violations) must have reached high-up ears. For we received a directive presently: "It is imperative that we quit using personal judgment." Now I grant that there have to be directives. But (I can say now) one of the frustrations of government work lay then, and probably lies now, in such hamstringing regulations. It always seemed to me that if you take the pains to find and to hire a trained employee to go into a field, no matter what the work, you owe it to him to give him the authority to make some decisions on his own to fit the facts in individual cases.

Instructions coming out of Washington used the word "imperative" all too freely. One of those instructions specified a one-half-inch needle. Now, I defy anyone to consistently make satisfactory injections with such a long needle, unless he chloroformed each cow in order to persuade her to hold still under the animal restraint equipment (or lack of equipment) we were forced to work with. I can see no disadvantage in allowing the veterinarian in charge to dictate his own needle length, as he will soon learn which length does the most satisfactory job. The first prerequisite, as I see it, in teaching a person responsibility is to give it to him.

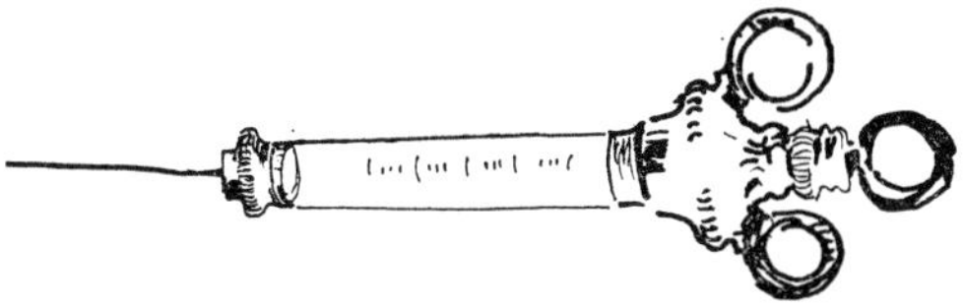

A case in point was the regulation that we could no longer work on Saturdays. In a country as sparsely settled as central Nevada, the only time any measurable source of help was available was on weekends. Most of the high school kids had grown up on ranches, where they had learned to ride and to rope; and the one big industry, Kennecott Copper, closed on weekends. These were our two labor sources. Frequently, it was Friday night before we learned whether we could get a crew together and this left no time for clearance with authorities in Washington. A rancher might call on Saturday, Sunday, or the Fourth of July to have his cattle tested and we felt obliged to go then.

Often, we took our own camper and Hazel looked after the records. Sometimes we took a friend along, to stamp the numbers on the backs corresponding to the numbers on the tubes containing blood. The important thing was to get the job done. Either you worked on weekends or you worked with the handicap of half a crew. Generally, to facilitate the business, we ran the samples in the ranch kitchen.

Some of the characters who helped us out were just that. One old codger by the name of Tom Thurmond claimed to be a relative to Will Rogers. His chin all but met his nose. I wouldn't venture a guess as to his age, but in roping he could well have competed with his famous kin. Thurmond never *whirled* a rope, he simply snaked it out and caught the animal by a front leg, and he never missed his target. "Which one you want?" he would ask, and before you could say "Will Rogers," he had it.

A stallion mauled Thurmond once and cut him up pretty badly, but the old man survived. One day not long after the accident Hazel encountered him in the basement of a store in Ely making a purchase of a suit of longjohns. The clerk accepted the old man's check with skepticism and took it to the manager. who declared, loud enough for the entire store to hear, that the check was a forgery. "Some horse killed the old coot more'n a month ago."

With a big herd and a small corral, we had to have sufficient help to keep the animals rounded up while we ran the blood samples to see whether we had a reactor. Otherwise, before the report got back from a lab, the animal might be miles away on the range. But we liked working with large herds. By testing one hundred and fifty animals in a herd of many thousands, the chance of getting at least one reactor was about ninety-five percent, even though the infection was only two percent.

One facet of brucellosis research has always interested me. The organism that causes the disease in cattle, where it has an affinity for uterine tissue, is also the guilty party in the ailment we call "fistulous withers" in horses, a condition characterized by the formation of passages or tubes through the tissues to the skin surface. The meaning of the word "fistulous" is "tubelike" or "tubular." We occasionally detected cases of fistulous withers in horses that worked among brucellosis-infected herds.

Even in Nevada, in the nineteen-sixties, we occasionally came along behind some salesman who claimed to have a brucellosis "cure." We found ranchers who swore by these remedies. If an animal diagnosed (by the salesman himself) as having the disease dropped her calf all right, the word went on to the next farm and the next.

One peculiarity concerning brucellosis lies in the fact that with hogs brucellosis is spread by the sire and the sow does not abort, she simply delivers a small litter. I recall a remark made by a diagnostician and researcher. When asked a question about porcine brucellosis, he replied, "One of the characteristics of abortion in hogs is that they do not abort."

In the *bovine* type of the disease, a male is rarely a factor. Earlier it was thought that brucellosis was a kind of venereal disease in animals, and sometimes we tested bulls, to humor the owner. We rarely found a reactor and testing bulls is not without its problems. Not many chutes are so constructed as to accommodate a large bull, and his hide is so thick that it is usually difficult to find a vein. On one occasion in my experience, *Bacterium brucella* showed up in an artificial insemination house and created quite an unexpected problem. But this was most unusual.

Too often, however, we did find that sales barns were clearing houses for diseased animals, not only for brucellosis but also for other conditions.

Finally, it was the combination of test and vaccination that brought brucellosis under control. We encountered opposition, but by and large the ranchers were more than cooperative and we had little complaint. No matter how worthwhile a program, you can always find someone who will take an opposite view just for the hell of it. Disease control (who can say, ever, that a disease has been "eradicated?") is often as difficult to promote for animals as for man. A suspicious faction of the public fought smallpox vaccination. Hundreds of groups still battle successfully against fluoridation. Federal veterinarians in Montana ran into strong opposition to vaccination of dogs and cats against rabies. Early tuberculosis testers were chased off Iowa farms with pitchforks. I have already recounted the difficulties faced by tick eradicators in the Southwest.

To be sure, we made mistakes. With brucellosis as with tuberculosis, there is always a margin of error and we were not supermen. And even though a cow may abort only one calf she can readily pass the disease along to heifers with which she associates, by the mere chance of switching her tail in a heifer's eye. Indeed, we found the tail switch in the eye one of the most potent of all the sources of infection.

When a testing program had been completed in a given area, the area was given a rating. The fact that east central Nevada was on a "free" status before I left the work gave me a good deal of satisfaction.

ACCOMPLICES

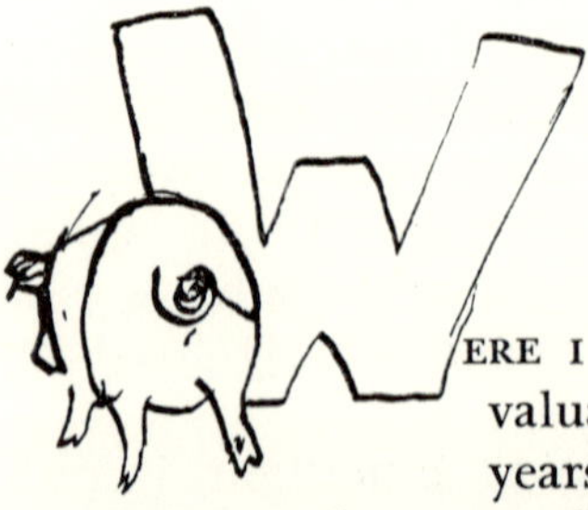

WERE I TO NAME all the people who lent invaluable assistance during my forty-odd years of work, the list would be long and it would include women (besides my wife Hazel) as well as laymen and vacationing students of veterinary medicine. I suppose a practitioner of human medicine could go it alone fairly well if necessary. But a veterinarian has to have assistance plenty of times. Although some animals prove so cooperative that you would swear they possessed so-called "human" intelligence, the majority naturally fear and resist treatment, as most children do.

During practice in Oklahoma, we kept a few cages out back of our combination office and living quarters for small animals left for treatment or observation. As I was out on call throughout most of the daylight hours, Hazel was frequently obliged to accept for my attention after supper some dog or cat brought in by its owner and to look after the animal until I got around to diagnosis and treatment.

We still laugh about a woman client from the country who rang the bell one afternoon in a considerable state of anxiety.

"The doctor's out on call," Hazel told her. "Is there something I can do?"

"Well, I don't know," the woman said. "I have two dogs in the car. The little female's mine. She was in season, you see, and I was keeping her in. But she got out. When I found her this male was attached. I couldn't get them separated, so I brought them both in, to see what the doctor could do."

Sure enough, Hazel told me, the two dogs occupied the back seat of the small sedan. After Hazel had explained the ways of dogs, she asked curiously how her caller had managed to get the pair corralled and loaded.

"Well, it wasn't easy," the woman admitted. "Becky . . . that's mine . . . wouldn't pay the slightest attention to me. I just had to get them cornered and pick them both up at once and get them into the car. Next time I'll buy a four-door."

One of Hazel's patients was a ruptured pig, and the finale was tragic as well as embarrassing. The owner called early in the morning of a busy day. I told him if he would bring the pig in and leave it I would try to operate that evening after supper.

About nine o'clock that evening I performed the operation, which didn't amount to much, put the pig back into the owner's sack in the garage, and asked Hazel to call the client to pick up the animal the next morning.

The farmer was late in coming. Finding that the pig had worked loose from the sack, Hazel closed the garage door. When the owner still had not come at midafternoon, she stepped into the garage to see how the patient fared. Like Eudora Welty's "Clytie," he had gone headfirst into a wooden ice cream tub half filled with water and had perished there.

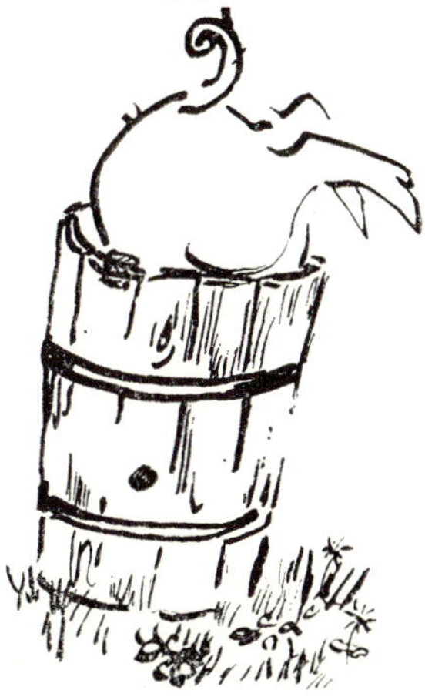

Largely, Hazel's share of the clients was confined to sick dogs and their owners. One dog fancier lived with her retarded daughter in a small house surrounded by kennels. The kennels housed at one time thirty-eight canines of assorted mixtures and sizes, and one or another of these animals was almost always ailing. Having no telephone, the owner summoned us by postal card, describing the symptoms in lay terms in her own colorful language.

If I had stopped at this particular doggery I had only to contact Hazel and then to hold the short wave transmitter outside the car in order to apprise her of my whereabouts. Hearing the yapping chorus, she would say, "I know. You're at Mrs. M's place."

I suppose these animals filled some psychological need, as did the fifteen Manchesters harbored and cherished by another female client. Better off than Mrs. M, she drove a pickup truck with accommodations for the dogs. One morning as I was about to start the day's rounds she brought in a young bitch she called Bessie that was about to deliver pups. The owner told me she feared complications.

I examined Bessie briefly. "She looks all right," I said. "It will just be a matter of time."

"All the same I'd like you to keep her here, Doctor. Just in case she has trouble."

"Well, there's a box in the garage," I said. "You may leave her there if you like."

She said, "I'd like to sit with her if you don't mind. This is her first confinement you know."

Hazel reported. "She wouldn't even come in for lunch. I took her a tray." Bessie delivered, normally, around five.

On Sunday evening, two days later, we returned from a visit to Hazel's father in Stanton. The red pickup stood in the driveway. This time the patient was "Violet." Violet proved to be in real trouble. In spite of all we could do, she didn't make it.

"Now, I want you to do a post mortem, Doctor," the owner told me. "To see what went wrong."

I have forgotten the results of the post. But I remember the call that came on the day following. "Did the doctor do an autopsy?"

"Yes, he did," Hazel said. "I'll get the results for you."

"That can wait," she said. "Did he put Violet back together?"

"Well, no . . . not exactly."

"I want him to do that," the caller said firmly. "I want to pickle her and take her back to Texas next summer, to bury in the garden."

She proved all too appreciative. She brought us food, most of it as unusable as a crock of rancid lard, and jelly so black and strong that we could neither eat nor identify the product. One day she called to ask whether we could use some dressed fryers.

"Thanks," Hazel said. "But we only use larger chickens."

"Then you wouldn't want these. They've had nothing to eat for six days. That's why I want to get rid of them."

One woman with a pet far advanced in years and hopelessly ill came to a wise decision, finally, painful I am sure, to ask me to put him to sleep. The method we used in such cases was to inject the animal with nembutal for sedation, followed by a quick injection of magnesium salts directly into the heart.

As a rule we experienced no difficulty. Although I knew he was in no pain, this one set up a stubborn and nervous barking following the injection, and kept it up throughout half the night. The following morning he had succumbed.

"Call Mrs. R," I told Hazel. "Tell her to come and get her dog." I reckoned she would want to bury him somewhere.

Mrs. R brought an elaborate casket, along with the dog's blanket and several toys. "But I don't want to take him with me now," she told Hazel. "Let him lie in state here today, just in case he should waken."

"About midmorning," Hazel told me, "I heard a sudden yipping noise. Completely undone, I dropped the vacuum and ran for the garage. To my enormous relief the dog still lay peacefully asleep." The sound, that mimicked the dog exactly, had come from baby Carol's room.

When I was in charge of the lab as an upperclassman I underwent a bizarre experience with one assistant and the use of nembutal as an anesthetic. A cat had been brought into the clinic for an operation. I asked my current helper, a kind of scatterbrained kid, to give the animal a shot of nembutal while I attended other chores.

"Put her on the scale," I instructed carefully. "Give her one cc for every five pounds of weight. Be sure it's exact weight and measurement."

When I walked into the room a short while later, the cat lay on the table. I took a second look. She was asleep all right, as flat as an unrisen pancake. Had she been near the edge, I think she would have literally flowed off the board.

Startled and suspicious, I asked my young helper, "How much nembutal did you give her?"

"Just what you told me," he bristled. "I gave her five cc's for every pound of weight."

I reckon she still may be asleep somewhere.

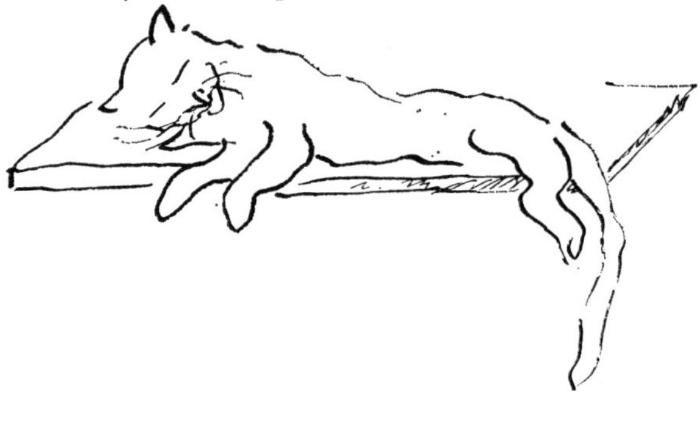

By the time we set up practice in Nebraska, Hazel had come to feel she knew a bit about veterinary medicine, as indeed she did. If a client called while I was away, she sometimes asked him to describe the symptoms so that she could pass the word along to me by short wave. Thus I could determine whether the case were an emergency and whether I had the proper instruments or medication.

When a farmer called to report a sick cow, Hazel asked how she acted.

He described the symptoms.

"Sounds like milk fever to me," she said. "Don't let her lie down flat. She'd be apt to bloat. You might put a blanket over her to keep her warm. I'll call the doctor."

I swung by as soon as I could. "How's the cow?" I asked when he came to the Jeep to meet me.

"She's got milk fever," he said. "Your wife told me."

"Well if my wife can diagnose by telephone," I said, not without pique, "I guess there's not much use in my looking at the cow. I'll just get the milk fever medicine."

We hired a good deal of help over the years and we also received a lot of assistance gratis. If you had a big job to do you could usually round up a crew of farm neighbors. As soon as Dean was old enough he went with me on calls, and he continued to work with me during weekends and vacations while he was in veterinary medical school.

I recall a winter day summons from a Mennonite preacher to help to pull a calf. The wind was blowing a gale. The thermometer stood at minus ten. The ground was covered by loose snow and snow whipped off drifts and blew across the fields and the road in clouds as dense as milk, a real Nebraska blizzard.

When Dean and I finally arrived at the client's place we were amazed to find the farmer shivering beside the fence in shirt sleeves. I could see the heifer across the field, a mass that I took to be the afterbirth dragging behind her.

"I guess she's already dropped her calf," I said. "She seems to be pulling her cleanings."

"No, she's not dropped her calf," the man of the cloth said, between chattering teeth. "And that's not her *cleanings* she's pulling. That's my *coat.* I tied the sleeves around the calf's neck to try to pull it, and she bolted and took the coat with her!"

On another occasion we received a call from a Bohemian

saying one of his cows had thrown her uterus. We cranked up the Jeep and hurried out.

We found the neighbors had been summoned and the situation pretty well under control. The menfolk followed the cow about the lot carrying a clean spread sheet, landing-net fashion, in anticipation of the organ's fall. The women were gathered in the kitchen, with coffee on the stove and kolaches ready.

Among the help one hog raiser had rounded up for a vaccination party was a burly chap who put on a performance I could scarcely credit. Picking up an eighty-pound pig by the hind legs he would give it a flip as easily as you would turn a rabbit and catch it by the front. He never missed.

"I know that guy," Dr. Person told me. "He's practically legendary. The story goes that he drove up to a country grocery down around Beemer one day and asked for salt."

" 'All the salt I've got is in three hundred-four hundred pound barrels in the cellar,' the grocer told him, 'and I don't have the help to bring it up.'

" 'I'll carry one of them up for you,' the fellow offered.

"The grocer snorted. 'Well, I'll give you all the salt you can carry in barrels up that stairwell.'

"That boy carried eight barrels up the grocer's steps, loaded them into his wagon, and drove off."

When sufficient routine jobs had accumulated, we would line up men and boys who knew something about roping and go from farm to farm. It wasn't quite as easy to find men in Nebraska who could throw a rope as it had been in Oklahoma, where every ten-year-old boy is something of an expert, but we could sometimes get a crew together on a weekend.

One Sunday an embarrassing thing happened. Having received several requests and rounded up a gang, we set out to castrate colts. At this particular farm we found the owner away. But I knew the colt, a big fellow weighing six or seven hundred pounds.

Using the mare as a mount, we managed, finally, to get the colt into the barn and get a rope on him. We had thrown a couple of hitches around a sill to snub him for the work at hand, when he reared suddenly, hit the rope, and bolted for the open door. That old barn collapsed as though it had been struck by an earthquake or a tornado.

The colt took off across the lot and tried to jump the barbed wire fence but became hopelessly entangled. When he could no longer move we decided to do the operation right there.

When we had finished, we doctored his wire cuts carefully and cut him loose. That was one time I really needed a crew. We had a barn to re-build before the owner got home, in addition to a fence-mending job.

One of our regular helpers was a funny, frail little fellow we called "Mousey." They used to say of Mousey that he only had a couple of red cells and they were bent. But he was willing and good-natured and he often made us laugh, an asset in any business.

One morning Mousey and I set out in the Jeep to vaccinate a few hogs. Inasmuch as we charged by the call, we encountered a (very) few clients who took advantage of the fact by saving up jobs, so that we might well spend a half day in one place. This saved *us* time, of course, but it could also be a trifle galling if we had a number of calls ahead. This one proved inclined to minimize the work by an elaborately casual approach. When we had finished vaccinating he asked us, offhand, if we wouldn't "just pinch a couple of young bull calves" while we were there. Before we had finished with that job, he had brought up "a little boar I'd like to have you cut."

We had to keep running back to the Jeep to change equipment. But at long last we had finished, or so we thought. We packed up our stuff and set out. As we were about passing the farmhouse, the owner came running down the driveway in pursuit, waving and shouting to us to "hold up!"

"Well, what the heck you reckon he wants now?" Mousey drawled as we slid to a stop. "We've done everything but grease the windmill."

When our daughter Marylin's husband Mike had finished school and come to work with me, the load was eased somewhat. If we had a number of calls he could go in one direction and I in another. As straw boss, I wasn't above dispatching Mike on some of the less desirable assignments.

One small herd on our list to test for brucellosis was owned by an ornery old goat with a slovenly wife and a house full of younguns. Rumor had it that the old man locked his wife upstairs when she had committed a misdemeanor. He even talked of buying a two-way radio for his tractor. "So's I can keep tab on the Missus."

"I'll let you take this one," I told Mike magnanimously.

"It's the house with the bedspring on the roof for a TV aerial. If you have trouble with him just mention the sheriff. He'll come around all right."

"Did you get any flak from old H?" I asked Mike at supper.

Mike grinned. "Not from H. From Mrs. H. She informed me in no uncertain terms that their cows didn't need testing. Said she'd drunk milk from that herd ever since she was married and had never had a single abortion. I couldn't doubt her word. There sat a kid on every fence post."

"Did you stay to dinner?"

He pulled a long face. "I didn't have any dinner. H. asked me to stay. We had just cut some bull calves as a kind of bonus job and he was gathering up the nuts to take to the house. I told him no, thanks, I'd had a late breakfast. He said o.k., that he'd planned to take me in to Pilger to eat at the restaurant but since I wasn't hungry we'd just skip it."

One spring day a widow who was trying to carry on on a hard scrabble farm following the death of her husband called to say her cows were going down. It had been a hard winter and we suspected malnutrition was the answer, but Mike offered to go out and see what he could do for her. "It was missmeal cramps all right," he told me. "I suggested she get in a load of hay and just let the animals at it."

The next day the widow called again. "I'm worried about that hay," she told Mike. "They all seem all right but one cow. She started to eat, and then fell dead beside the stack. Do you think it could have been the hay that killed her, Doctor?"

"Well, in a way," he said soothingly. "But I wouldn't worry about the others if I were you. I reckon it was the hay she didn't get that killed her."

One Christmas after Mike came we pulled a dirty trick on Hazel. As superintendent of the local Sunday school, she was supposed to round up a Santa Claus for the Christmas program at the church. She had tried her best to coerce me into doing the job and had put together a costume that more or less fitted. But I kept putting her off. I'm not much good at the kind of palaver a Santa ought to have, and I felt that even the youngest would know my voice. She had tried, too, to persuade Mike, but he, too, had put her off.

When the night of the program rolled around she was still without a character to fill the role and was still after us. Mike, who is a good deal heavier than I, argued that the costume wouldn't fit. We had had a hard day and were both tired. Animals are as apt to get sick at Christmas time as at any other. In a country as cold as Nebraska they're more apt to come down with something in the winter. We might well have to go out on call.

"Grouse, grouse," she said. "I'm leaving. The suit's in there on the bed and it's big enough for either one of you. Mike can just wear fewer pillows. When I shake those sleigh bells one of you had better show up, or there'll be no Christmas dinner tomorrow!"

"Mike," I said after she had gone, "do you reckon we could find another Santa Claus suit?"

"Sure," he said. "I know a fellow who's got one."

"Let's both show up."

When the signal sounded I popped in through the back door. At the same moment Mike entered the front. But we dispensed with the usual jollity. We met in the center aisle and started yelling at each other. The kids took sides. I thought Hazel would kill us both. But everybody else seemed to like the show, and the story made the Omaha paper.

Dave was a game enough youngster, but he had never handled animals. He was on hand one evening when a tomcat was brought in to be altered. With a male kitten, we never used an anesthetic, feeling that the needle was actually more painful than the pinching. We simply put the cat into a gunny sack, an old-fashioned but safe method. Following one such operation I turned the cat over to Dave to take back to the kennel where he was to be held for the owner. Dave took the sack but was a good while putting in a reappearance. His hands and arms were crisscrossed with bloody scratches.

"Good Lord, Dave," I asked. "What happened?"

"Nothing much, Doc," he said, getting down the iodine. "I got him out of the sack all right. But then he started to run before I could put him down."

Two of our most satisfactory helpers were women without any previous training in the field. One was Mrs. Bill (Marge) Holland, the wife of a client. Bill called one morning to ask if I could come out and look at a little sow that was about to farrow.

The little sow was in trouble all right. "If we just had someone with a hand small enough to pull that first pig," I said, "I think she could bring the others."

"Could Marge do it?"

"Would Marge do it?" I doubted whether Marge had ever seen a sow farrow, let alone acted as midwife. But I knew she was a very thrifty woman. "We might tell her the sow will die unless she has help," I said, "and there's nothing either of us can do." I wasn't sure but that this was the case.

Marge gave us an outraged negative.

"Well, then," Bill said, "you can mark her down in your books as a loss, along with the loss of what her pigs would bring."

She thought that over. "Oh, all right," she said finally. "If Doc will tell me what to do."

I've never seen a neater job of porcine obstetrics, nor a midwife prouder of her accomplishment. Many times afterward I had occasion to call upon Marge for help. "I'm going out to So-and-so's place, Marge," I would tell her. "He's got a sow that's about to farrow. Put on your overalls and I'll be by to pick you up." She never failed me.

Another female assistant was Margaret Young of McGill, Nevada, the wife of the Kennecott manager. Having heard me say one day that I needed someone to number the cattle as they came through the chute for vaccination, she said, "I'll go, if you'll tell me what to do." (The numbering was done with aluminum paint.)

She did a bang-up job. Furthermore, she appeared to have a great time. When I stopped in at a ranch one day and found a shortage of hands I remarked to the owner, "Well, I think I know a woman who will help. I'll call Mrs. Young over at McGill."

"You don't mean Mrs. Roy Young?"

"Sure," I said. "She's helped us out before."

He stared in disbelief. "Good Lord," she's the Kennecott manager's wife!"

Nevada was one place where we always seemed to be shorthanded. Hazel went along to keep the records. But I always had to trust to find some help in the vicinity. At one ranch, I recall, we made use of a squat little Indian woman, wife of one of the ranch hands. Her job, too, was to mark the animals. The cows had been going through the chute in good shape, when the line came to a sudden stop.

The little woman appeared to be arguing hotly with her husband, who was helping to chute. I called out, "What seems to be the trouble, John?"

"Maybe you can straighten it out, Doc. She's bound an

eleven is wrote with three ones. I claim it's only two."

Howard was a slow, shy youngster, but good help. When we worked around home he took his noon meal with us. One day Hazel called us in to lunch. "Now, there's only ham and beans today," she said as we sat down. "Anyone who doesn't like either will just have to go elsewhere."

Howard arose gravely from the table. "I'll see you at one o'clock, Doc," he told me. Taking up his hat, he set off up the street toward the restaurant.

We found no dearth of self-help. So long as they weren't just self-starters who expected us to bail them out of a bungled job, we didn't mind. We had plenty to do and were always glad to give instructions over the telephone or otherwise so long as we knew the client would do as he was told. Some of these calls were pretty far-fetched.

Late one night a woman called me out of a sound sleep to ask about her cat. "He has a sore on his leg," she told me. "I just wanted to ask if it would be all right to give him penicillin."

"Well, that depends," I said. "Check your container and see whether the penicillin is combined with streptomycin." Some cats won't tolerate the latter.

I could hear voices in the background. There seemed to be some kind of argument afoot. She returned to the telephone.

"The label don't mention streptomycin," she said. "As a matter of fact, it don't say anything about penicillin either."

I was thoroughly awake now, and a trifle disgruntled. "Well, where did it come from? What was it used for?"

"It's something we got from Dr. X for a bloated calf a year or so ago."

"Well I reckon anything that's good for a bloated calf ought to help a cat with a sore leg," I told her. "But don't call me if it kills him."

One day a frantic call came from a good client whose hogs we had vaccinated against erysipelas. He himself had given the hogs a booster shot, he said in great distress, and had then made the discovery (as has many a hapless soul) that he had picked up the wrong bottle. He had injected the animals with a forty percent solution of lindane, kept on the barn shelf to treat for lice and scab. To make matters worse, one of the victims was a purebred York sow he had borrowed. He had given her a total of forty cc's. His own Hampshire had been injected with eighty cc's.

I came on the run. The animals stood with their heads down, drooling as though from an awful taste. They all had a little swelling behind the ears. The owner followed me from one to the other asking, "Will they die, Doc?" He was at the same time funny and pathetic.

"Lord, I don't know," I told him finally. "You've vaccinated more hogs with lindane than I ever did."

The hogs slobbered for two days, and declined to eat. But they all recovered. Most of them went to market presently and the meat passed inspection. But I couldn't help wondering a bit about the flavor of the bacon.

As our two daughters grew older I took them along sometimes on calls. Marylin, the eldest, had finished nurses' training before she married Mike and was a good deal of help. The youngest, Carol, was just a kid. But she liked to think of herself as indispensable. Occasionally when we went out for the evening we left her to tend office and to answer the telephone. On one such evening a good client came in and asked for me.

"He's not here," he reported Carol told him. "But if you've come to pay the bill I can take the money."

I suppose Carol was around ten when I was called out one day to treat a cow for some ailment. Carol had a friend visiting for the day and I asked the two girls to ride along.

The cow was milling about the lot along with a few other animals, including an unpleasant looking bull that seemed both mean and mad, and I instructed the girls to stay in the car.

When I had finished treating the cow the owner walked to the car with me. "I think she'll be all right," I told him. "Is she due to calve soon?"

"In another month or so," he said.

As soon as we were underway, Carol asked, "Was that cow pregnant, Dad?"

"Well, yes, I guess she is," I said.

She settled back. "Well, no wonder that bull was mad!"

Our son Dean had gone with me on calls from the time he was a little fellow and he had learned to ride and to rope. During his years in veterinary school our practice in Nebraska was heavy; and although we lived some two hundred miles from the school, he often came for weekends, bringing along a friend or two from the college. These boys not only learned a bit in a practical sense, they proved good help when help was sorely needed and difficult to come by.

One skill we attempted to teach these youngsters who came to us from time to time as helpers was how to throw a rope. We encountered practicing veterinarians who had never been on a horse, and most of them managed, I reckon. But I do not know how I would have made out in either the Oklahoma Panhandle or central Nevada had I not known how to ride and rope. In either area, almost every ten-year-old boy could lasso a calf from on horseback, and I would have been considerably embarrassed. "You don't really have to be a cowboy in order to be a veterinarian," I heard a young practitioner remark once, "but it sure as hell helps to be."

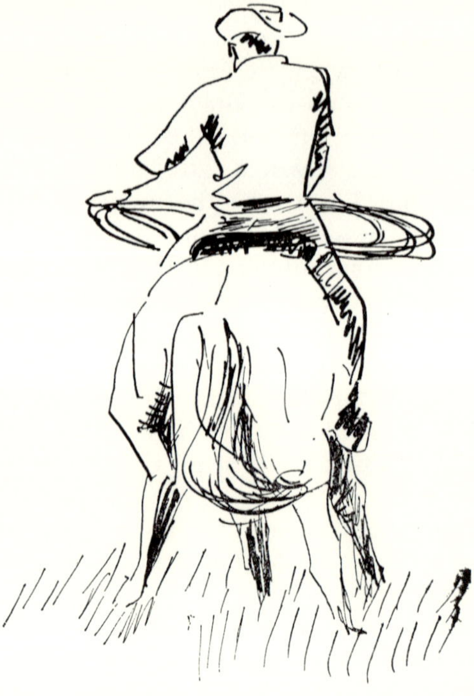

I remember a morning when one serious-minded student came home with Dean for a weekend when we had nothing on the docket. He kept saying, "I hope something turns up." We were dawdling over breakfast around nine o'clock when the telephone rang.

From then on we were deluged with calls. We pulled calves, vaccinated, cleaned cows, sewed cuts, injected hogs, extracted teeth. As a finale, late that evening, we were called out to castrate a show mule. A big animal, he was as comical as any creature I ever saw. He would lie down at a command, roll over on his back with feet in air and play dead, or gently administer to his trainer a well-placed kick. Our visiting student was worn out but elated. He made a good veterinarian. Like a lot of young people nowadays (indeed, as we were) he was married while still in school.

"Boy, was I ever dumb about animals," his wife told Hazel. "Bob went to the office one evening to spay a female dog and asked me to go along. That operation was certainly an eye opener. I thought all he was going to do was to sew up the little opening below the tail."

ASSORTED CUTS

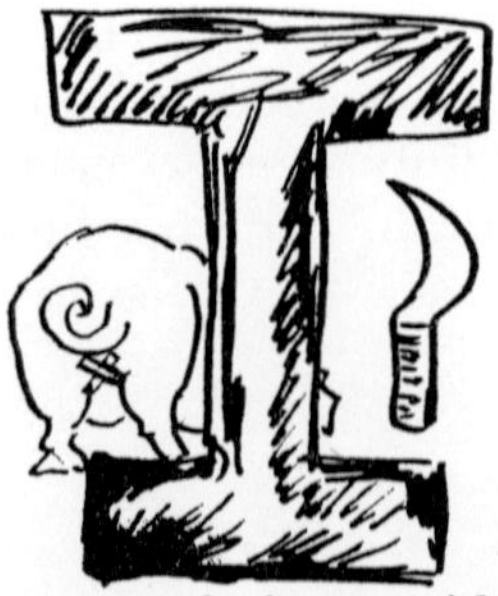

I DON'T KNOW what present-day veterinary schools call the testes. Most farmers and ranchers I encountered said "nuts," just as many of them said "spaded" for "spayed." Had we said anything save "cut" and "nuts" for "castrated" and "testes," a good many farmers wouldn't have known what we were talking about or would have thought we were trying to put on airs.

Among most cowboys the bit of meat removed in castration, especially from a young animal, was considered a delicacy. In the Oklahoma Panhandle the boys who helped with the roundup and the chuting threw the nuts into the branding fire and ate them on the spot. Hazel had a special recipe. She put the glands into a skillet in order to simmer the water off, added salt and pepper, poured condensed cream of mushroom soup over the lot, and slid them into a moderate oven for 30 minutes to tenderize. We used lamb, pork, and calf testes. We rarely bothered with testes from older animals, as they were apt to be strong and tough.

My own strictly amateur career as a vet began with a calf castration on a muddy day following a spring rain when I was ten or eleven years of age. Because of the press of spring work, Dad had chosen a day too wet to get into the fields as a time to cut and to earmark the spring calves. As my brothers Charles and Myron and I corraled the little herd and put the first calf into the chute, Dad sat patiently whetting his pocket knife on a whetstone. When he had finished, he arose and, to my astonishment, handed the knife to me.

"You do the cutting today, Willet," he directed. "My hands are too shaky for this job."

I took the knife, uncertain, and more than a little frightened, and did exactly as he told me. The fact that no animal died (so far as I can recall) as a result of my quackery, I attribute not to my skill but to sheer luck and to his patient instruction.

I do recall a battle with screw worms that resulted from a bit of bad advice on the part of a cattle buyer by the name of Haz Reed who operated a retail meat market, then called a "butcher shop," in Coffeyville, Kansas. In those days of simpler and smaller operations, cattle went from farm to feed yard to abattoir to outlet shop without changing ownership, thus eliminating middlemen. Reed drove into our place on a hot August day to take away some fifteen or twenty head of cattle he had purchased, and found Dad lamenting the fact that he had been too busy in the spring to castrate the bull calves and was afraid to do the job so late in the season.

"But there's no danger, Bill," Reed assured him, "as long as the calves aren't weaned yet. The cows will keep the wounds licked clean and no nits will hatch."

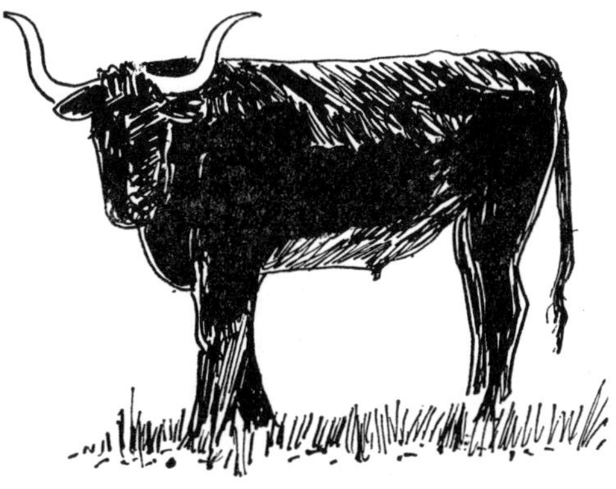

As a rule Dad did not much trust cattle buyers, but he had a good deal of confidence in Reed, who had never cheated him. We would cut the calves the following day, he decided. I especially remember that hot August and the long sweltering weeks afterward because of the screw worms. Every calf we castrated became infected, and one died. We fought the infestation in the only way we knew. We poured chloroform into the wounds and held pads of cotton over the mess until the larvae were asphyxiated. Then we treated the wounds with pine tar. But the larvae kept hatching. It has often occurred to me that this was certainly one of the times when we should have invested the two or three dollars a veterinarian would have charged for a call.

I don't know how efficacious the pine tar was or whether it was any good at all. But it was the only remedy we knew. Later, a product with a fish oil base proved effective. In the Oklahoma Panhandle nearly all of the cowboys carried a cresylic ointment for use in case they came across an infested animal on the range.

While we are on the unpleasant subject, I will digress to say that it is not uncommon to find both screw worms and maggots in the same wound. One of my pet peeves when I worked for the government in the field had to do with our instructions to send specimens of larvae to the laboratory before we could say which of the two we had found. Any ten-year-old boy who has been around livestock to any extent can distinguish between the two. Maggots live on *dead* tissue; screw worms go for *live* tissue. At one time an effort was made to "clean up" wounds by the *introduction* of the former.

Some day, hopefully, animals will not be subjected to this nasty infestation. The present experiment of distributing sterilized male blowflies as a method of control looks promising. That the deer population in the southern part of the United States (especially south Texas and Arizona) is on the increase, authorities say, seems an indication that the program is working.

The biggest and the wildest nut-cutting operation I ever supervised was in the Oklahoma Panhandle for a mule buyer by the name of Bill Harrison who had worn out a Dodge truck driving around to buy up mule colts. When he had assembled some three hundred colts he asked me to come out and clip off some warts and castrate the males. One Sunday I rounded up a crew and drove out.

Those mules were as wild as any coyotes. Having looked the lot over, we built a chute out from the barn door, long enough to hold two mules and on a slope, reasoning that when the gate was opened the animals would go forward and down. Bill's son Frank and a cowpuncher named Pinky Munson, a pair of real cowhands with plenty of grit, were on hand to help with the job. To throw the mules, we used two sets of casting harness. A mule has a long thin head and can edge out of a harness, so we kept a man at the head end to guard against this exigency. Once a colt was down, we tied the right hind leg in order to hold him and to protect ourselves from a lambasting. Still, by the time we had finished with those rascals, Frank and Pinky had hardly a stitch of clothing left intact. But they never let a colt go until we were through with him.

That day, we castrated ninety-two colts of varying ages. I always preferred to castrate two-year-old horse colts, but we sometimes cut a mule as old as five. The mules were branded at the same time and we kept the knives disinfected in a copper kettle of boiling water over the branding fire. For some reason of his own, Dad had always taken out the left testis first, and for no other reason than this I followed the same routine.

We had thrown more than a hundred mules to castrate and to clip warts that day, at fifty cents a head, and I was growing tired and a trifle edgy. When I ran out of towels and had to go back to the house, the rancher's wife, who was probably growing a trifle edgy herself, began to complain. "You didn't bring nothing much along with you, did you Doctor?" she told me sarcastically as she threw down the wanted towels.

"Yes, Ma'am, I did," I told her. "You may have noticed at noon that I brought along a good appetite."

Occasionally we met with a small accident. Once a mule struck the knife and I got a pretty bad cut. On a day I remember as being about the longest day I ever practiced, I sustained a scalp wound from a kick on the head, even though I always wore a hat. Driving home, half asleep, long after dark, I encountered a washed-out bridge and had to drive ten miles out of my way in order to negotiate the river.

One big cutting job in Nebraska had a funny aftermath. On a Sunday in June, a good hog man by the name of Neal Coy called to say he had around two hundred 150-pound boars in need of castration. A big job of this sort was always a kind of challenge as well as a temptation to grandstand a bit. They used to say back in hand corn husking days that a good cornpicker could keep an ear of corn in the air. Likewise, in my business, they sometimes said a good veterinarian faced with a big job of castration could "keep a nut in the air."

Having heard of the call from Coy, an antique dealer named Anderson who always operated the firemen's lunch stand at the annual Fourth of July picnic and celebration asked me if he could ride along to Coy's place.

I told him, "Sure." We were always glad to get any extra help available.

On the way out, Anderson explained that this looked like a good opportunity to pick up some nuts to freeze and serve at the firemen's dance. I didn't tell him how big these boars were, but I resolved to eat my lunch elsewhere.

Anderson thought he had run into a real bonanza. By the time we had finished with the job he had a ten-gallon cream can and a five-gallon pail completely filled with nuts.

On the night of the dance, he hailed me as I was passing the firemen's stand, where he was dishing out a kind of loose hamburger he called a "sloppy Joe."

"I'm snowed under, Doc," he told me. "Would you mind helping out for a bit?"

He had a two-burner hot plate going, with a kettle on each burner, but only one flame was lit. I rolled up my sleeves and lit the fire under the second kettle and started waiting on trade. Presently Anderson noticed what I was doing.

"Hey! No!" he said. "Turn out that fire, Doc!"

"And serve this stuff lukewarm?"

"We have to," he said earnestly. "This hot kettle here is made with beef. It's for the regular trade. The other's made from those boar nuts and it's for the drunks. As long as it's lukewarm they won't know what they're eating. But heat it up and it tastes like an old boar smells."

Occasionally we performed an operation for cryptorchidism, a word meaning undescended testes. A testis left in the belly of a meat animal, it was believed, gave meat a bad flavor. We performed this operation on horses and mules as well.

One day a storekeeper at Woodward, Oklahoma, called to say that his son-in-law who lived on the storekeeper's farm had a mule that was killing calves. "I think he's got a nut in his belly," he explained, "and that's what's making him mean. I wonder if you'd drive out and have a look at him."

Instead, I found a five-year-old mule that had never been castrated, and I went ahead and did the job. After a week or so, I had a second call. "You know that mule you cut, Doc?" he said. "It didn't do a damned bit of good. He's still killing calves."

All I could say in my own defense was that I had tended to an operation that needed doing. I hadn't guaranteed to cure the mule of cussedness.

A DISSERTATION UPON LIVE PORK

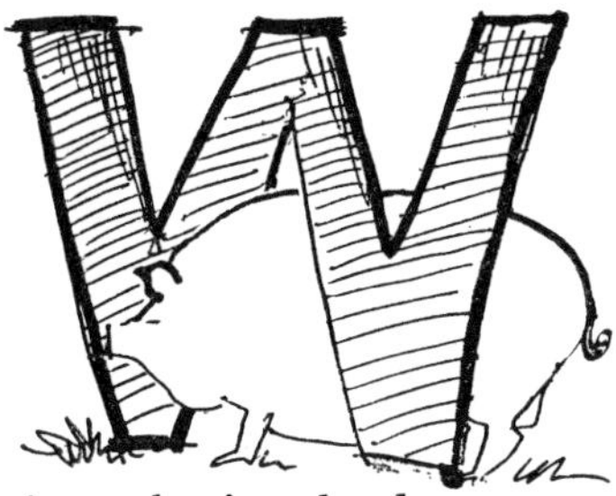

WHEN the late Henry Ford made a prediction that our food would one day come in pellet form, cutting short the involved process of raising plant to raise animal to feed man, he was dismissed as a crackpot.

A few years ago I encountered a setup for raising hogs that half inclines me to the belief that we may someday find a method of shoveling protein into one end of a hopper and taking sausage out the other, and so eliminate the hog. Having done away with the hog, they just may stuff a goodly percentage of the country's veterinarians into the hopper, too. Swine are susceptible to more kinds of diseases more often than any other creature I know.

The above-mentioned method of raising porkers seemed neither humane nor much fun for the hog, but I reckon it was good economics, which seems to justify about any practice of production these days. I suppose the life of the force-fed goose whose liver is developed for paté de fois gras would have some parallel. And I am bound to admit (if sanitation means anything to a hog, which I doubt) that these were kept immaculately clean.

The animals stood in individual stalls in an air-conditioned building. They could lie down and stand up, but they could not turn around. Each wore a collar attached to a foot-long chain that was in turn fastened to a ring in the slatted floor. Droppings were flushed away by turning paddle wheels below in a stream of water.

At precisely timed intervals a liquid, measured diet consisting of whey and grain flowed through a clean trough within reach of the hog's snout. When he had attained a given weight, I was told, ranging from two hundred and ten to two hundred and twenty pounds or as deemed desirable, he was released from bondage, sent up a ramp to a truck, to be carted away with his fellows to a slaughter house. During his lifetime his feet never touched earth. His pupils having no time to adjust to outside light during his brief exposure to daylight on the ramp, he was almost totally blind. But of course he had no use for sight. The scene made me feel old, and useless, and more than a little sad.

That a hog can think up more ways to die than the veterinary profession can think up means to save him is as much truth as proverb. But it occurs to me that man, as a civilized animal, has done something to the species over the centuries that he had no right to do to a fellow mammal. In the interest of meat and fat for ingestion by the human species, the porker has been changed into a creature with less than a third the lung capacity per pound of weight enjoyed by every other domestic animal. As a consequence he suffers endlessly from diseases of the respiratory system.

Consider the wild boar. Endowed with great strength, long legs for speed, vicious tusks for self-defense, and ferocity when at bay, this rather magnificent animal possessed a snout for rooting his sustenance from the earth and could hold his own under almost any circumstance. Partially domesticated around 2900 B.C., he was used as a scavenger, no thought being given as yet to his use as food for man. But then, as every schoolboy knows, came the story of the first roast pork.

Following this discovery the hog was rapidly domesticated. He was penned in a small area. His food was poured into a trough. He waddled forward to eat, and waddled back to his mudhole to lie down. He had no reason to exercise, nor did man wish him to do so. Over the years, as his lungs decreased in size their capacity diminished. He ate with head down, breathing close to the earth. His legs shortened. From generation to generation he was plagued by chronic viruses. The only requirement made of him was that he grow fat.

When, finally, a class of urbanites nearly as sedentary as the hog himself came into being, his layers of fat lost their popularity. By means of diet control, he was slimmed down to leaner meat. When cholesterol was "discovered" man turned to making the hog's corn into corn oil, to replace lard, a short cut that eliminated the hog as a producer of fat.

I do not know how disease-susceptible the present-day wild boar may be nor how far our own responsibility goes for the ills his flesh is heir to. Men involved in meat inspection maintain that the instructions of Moses and later prophets concerning pork had an intelligent scientific basis, that the parasite trichina that causes trichinosis when ingested may even then have been at work.

From the standpoint of the digestive system and type of food consumed, man and hog are a good deal more closely related than are cow and man. Perhaps a lesson for man, too, lies along the road down which the hog has journeyed through a few thousand years. The lack of lung capacity has made the hog painfully vulnerable to temperature changes. Because a hog does not sweat he must depend upon his inadequate lungs for air conditioning (unless, to be sure, he is so "fortunate" as to live out his span under the controlled situation above described).

When we went through a prolonged period of one hundred three- and one hundred four-degree temperatures in the Middlewest hogs died faster than the rendering trucks could gather them. During our professional rounds we used often to encounter one of these salvage men, a Frank Spangler. "Stop following us, Frank," we begged him. "Go follow another veterinarian. This makes us look bad."

When the time came that detergents all but eliminated the use of soaps made from animal fats, the rendering truckers began to charge for picking up dead animals. Of course some animal fat is still used in explosives. But we have encroached upon the prerogative of the cow by introducing margarine, imitation sweet cream, imitation sour cream, even imitation milk. Lately in a supermarket we came across a product labeled "imitation ham." We have all encountered imitation hamburgers, made from soybeans. Is it too far-fetched to wonder whether both hog and cow may one day vanish from the scene?

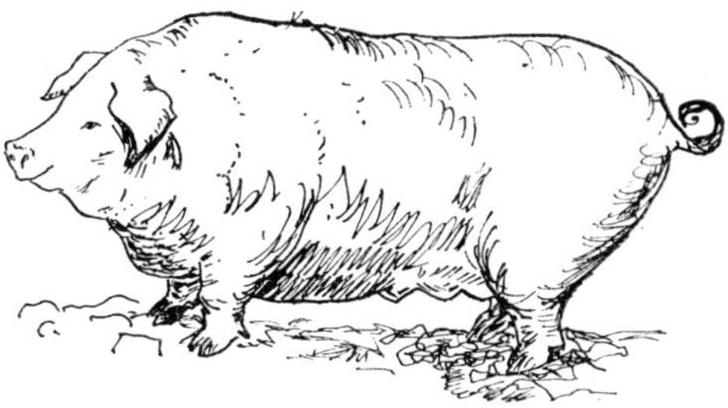

In hog country, many urban areas sooner or later got into some kind of controversy about hogs and garbage disposal. Both in and out of the service, I sometimes landed in the middle of one of these rows. If it came to taking sides, I usually found myself on the side of the hog. In my opinion the average household garbage is unfit for hogs and the hog man is actually rendering a service to the public when he condescends to gather such and not feed it to his herd.

Many a battle has been fought at city hall over this issue. Once it was believed that the nematode *Trichinella spiralis* found in the intestines and muscle tissue of hogs, came because the animals ate rats. Quite a furor arose when an Illinois researcher proved beyond a shadow of a doubt that the condition resulted from hogs having literally eaten hogs, in the form of uncooked pork scraps in unprocessed household garbage.

The discovery resulted in stringent regulations. Garbage fed to hogs must be cooked as thoroughly as pork for human consumption. Both in the vicinity of army camps where garbage was in use as hog feed, and later, in Nevada, my job included a periodic temperature check to see that the mess was being thoroughly sterilized.

In Pocatello, Idaho, during the war we engaged in a little war of our own that had to do with hogs and garbage. The mess officer ran a "consolidated mess" and did a good job of it. He had to be ready to feed a flying crew whenever they came in from overseas or across country, no matter what the hour.

The army held a garbage contract with a local hog raiser that stipulated "no coffee grounds nor glass." The hog man was in his rights of course. The law was on his side. But the lieutenant was a conscientious man. And so I was surprised when the farmer reported a loss of hogs and blamed coffee grounds and glass in the garbage. When a directive went out to the effect that if any more hogs died the lieutenant was in trouble, I drove out on a Sunday morning to do a little investigating on my own.

As I looked across a creek that ran through the hog yard I could see that several hogs, presumably dead, did indeed lie about on the other side. I contacted the owner of the herd to ask why the animals had not been removed from the premises.

He was something less than cooperative. He told me in a surly manner that he couldn't get in after them and that all of the sick hogs over there had died. I called the federal office in

Boise with a request that they send out a veterinarian to look the animals over.

He named the death cause as erysipelas. But you do not get a one hundred percent death loss from erysipelas. Suspicious now, I posted one of the dead animals. They had died of cholera. Nor were we long in learning the probable source. The owner was feeding the garbage *raw*. Out of a herd of five hundred, he lost eighty head, a considerable blow. But I was happy to be able to write a report to keep the lieutenant from being busted.

In a case of this kind you can always draw an argument to the effect that the animals a man owns are his own business. This is not quite the case. If you have diseased animals your neighbor has as much right to be protected as he has to be protected from human contagion. The fact that the government could step in with an animal quarantine was especially important during the war. The country simply couldn't afford an epidemic, of whatever nature.

In the Nevada area I was surprised to find that the chief source of garbage fed to hogs was neither household nor restaurant but the local food stores. I saw feeders' storerooms literally filled with stale cake mixes, broken boxes of pancake flours, cereals, Bisquick, every sort of prepared and semi-prepared food. Some of these smelled delicious in the cooking vats.

The only hog man I ever knew who made a garbage contract pay and pay well lived in the Nevada area. A man named Vittorini picked up garbage at both restaurants and feed stores. Several of these former were short order houses that served big steaks to cattlemen. Often half the steak was left on the plate. Those hogs lived pretty high on the cow.

My job there, too, included periodic stops to test Vittorini's cooking vats for temperature. I never found him in violation. He knew how to use garbage. The general run being too "sloppy" to make a good diet, he threw a bushel or so of barley into each vat, to serve as a roux.

One day my boss at Ely asked how I was getting along with Vittorini. "Oh, we get along first rate," I told him. "He always hauls out a jug of his home-made wine."

"Makes his own wine, eh?"

"I reckon he makes it out of the fruit he picks up behind the stores."

I thought Jack would surely know I was joking. But he

went along the next time I went out to Vittorini's place. When he lifted the lid off one of Vittorini's wine barrels a funny look came over his face and he said, "Come here, Doc."

The brew was topped with cut-up oranges, segments of grapefruit, and pieces of lemon, all floating on the surface.

When Vittorini's hogs developed sore feet, he sent for me. Soreness in an animal's feet is always something to be investigated because of the threat of hoof-and-mouth disease. We tended too, to think of vesicular emphysema, which can be mistaken for the former in some stages.

This time too, the garbage proved responsible. But the soreness came from the hogs walking about on sharp steak bones. Another hazard Vittorini's hogs had to contend with was restaurant cutlery. During bouts of inspection, we resurrected literally hundreds of knives, forks, spoons, even pitchers, cups, and plates that had gone out through the back doors and into the garbage cans.

Whether in human or veterinary pathology, the word "cholera" has a dreadful sound. As a boy, I remember hearing my folks talk about certain babies in the area sick or dying of *cholera infantum* and of certain older people suffering from *cholera morbus*. Periodically, some farmer's hogs started dying of a sickness diagnosed as cholera, and all of the neighbors gave the place a wide berth. I still shake a little to recall a Sunday morning watermelon stealing excursion on the part of myself, my brother Charles, and our friend Chet Reardon, to the patch of a neighbor who had lost a number of hogs to the disease, which all hog raisers thought, then, to be highly contagious.

Actually, cholera is a contagious disease. But we know now that it is generally spread by direct contact between the animals, not by carrier, on clothing or shoes. We had chosen a Sunday morning for the invasion because we knew that the neighbor, L, and his family would be at church then. Purportedly because I was the smallest in stature and so the least visible, the others chose me for the honor of visiting the patch and bringing out the melons, assuring me that they would stand watch. I objected on the grounds that I was wearing a white shirt.

"I'll give you mine," Chet offered generously, peeling out of the garment. "Bring all you can. We'll wait in the rock quarry."

After considerable reconnoitering and thumping, I chose two fine specimens and began the long crawl back along the hedge fence, pushing the booty ahead of me as a tumblebug pushes his ball of dirt. But either our timing was at fault or I had wasted too much time at the choosing. For, long before I had reached the safety of the quarry I heard the rattle of wheels as L's carriage turned in at the drive.

Embracing a melon under each arm, I hugged the earth while L set about unhitching and unharnessing his team. Precarious as was my own position, that of my collaborators in crime proved even less fortuitous. In their haste to escape being seen, they had abandoned me to my probable fate and had dived into the rock quarry, only to find themselves cheek by jowl with thirty or forty ripely dead and deadly ripe hogs, dumped into the quarry after they had died of cholera. For nearly an hour, Chet and Charlie were pinned down (in the term of soldiers in combat) while I waited, also "pinned down," for the farmer and his family to enter the house, making it safe for me to worm my way back to my miscreant companions.

The horrible stench was only a part of their dilemma. Chet being considerably larger than I, my shirt failed to cover enough of his back and arms to prevent a bad burn from the searing sun above the unshaded quarry. Rivaling the inside of the ripe melons in color, from both sunburn and displeasure over my belated arrival, the pair greeted me with highly ungrateful epithets . . . considering the unshared risk I had recently taken.

Afraid to confess to Dad, we watched our own hogs secretly and uneasily and avoided them as completely as possible. That neither the Reardon animals nor ours came down with cholera, we regarded as some kind of special dispensation.

As a general rule, Dad kept only sufficient hogs for our winter meat, and so we experienced little porcine trouble. When a sow took a notion to consume her own young, as our sows did sometimes, we knew nothing to do save to take the young away as soon as they were born and to get rid of the sow as an unfit mother. After I entered practice, we thought we had learned a thing or two about this strange obsession, but we never really found anything much in the way of prevention or panacea. A mother sow and a mother cat seem to have this in common: If either is disturbed during delivery, the work may come to a halt, or she may set about to deliberately devour her own offspring.

EXPECT THE UNEXPECTED

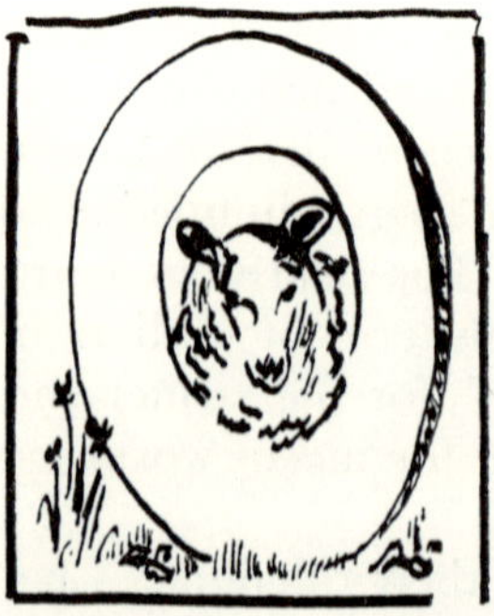

ONE DAY during my early practice in the Oklahoma Panhandle I encountered an occupational hazard, in the shape of a big white bull with the longest and meanest set of horns I have ever seen sprout from an animal's head, plus a disposition to match.

To make matters worse, the owner, an eccentric bachelor, was extraordinarily fond of his pet and proud of his great rack. But when the monster attacked a mule, puncturing a lung and leaving a nasty wound in the mule's side, the owner sent for me and remarked regretfully, "I reckon it's about time to dehorn him, Doc."

"Well, all right, if you say so," I agreed reluctantly. "But let's see to the mule first. He's lost a good deal of blood." Dehorning that big bastard was one job I didn't relish and I wanted to postpone as long as possible.

I sewed up the mule's wound as best I could, and, knowing that he was bound to roll in the dirt, tied a wide bandage securely around his middle. Meanwhile, as though he knew his turn was coming next and as though he were just itching to get at me, the bull watched belligerently from beyond the fence. Each time I looked in his direction he seemed to grow a little bigger.

Having finished with the mule, I sized up the situation. There wasn't a chute on the place, and anyway it would have taken an oversize one to hold him. I always carried a throw rope, but I knew he would go through that as though it were so much household twine. Rummaging in the car, I came up with a set of casting harness. When I came back, the owner had produced a dull-looking saw and stood beside the fence talking soothingly to his pet.

"Do you suppose we can get this on him?" I asked. "He's not going to like this much."

"I know," he said. "Poor boy. I can put a little grain in his box in the shed, I reckon."

After he had finally coaxed the big brute inside by using a bucket of corn and a lot of gentle persuasion, I hung the casting harness over the door. Keeping a wary eye on the by-now suspicious gentleman, I snugged the end of the contraption around a sturdy cottonwood tree, and stepped back.

We didn't have long to wait. As though aware suddenly that he was being had, the bull hooked one of his trophies inside the grain box, ripping the box to splinters, and then whirled and came ploughing out through the doorway with the energy of an express train at full throttle. The moment he hit the casting harness I pulled the rope taut around the tree. The board fence went down as though it had been a line of standing dominoes. But the rope held. I pulled his big head over against the tree so I could get at him and set to work.

Aware that the owner was watching uneasily as the animal began to make choking sounds, I felt obliged to explain, "If we don't half kill him he'll kill us you know."

When the second horn fell, finally, I cautiously untied the rope and got out of the way, having previously mapped the best evacuation route. The bull was fighting mad by that time, and I couldn't say that I blamed him any. He was spouting blood from both horn sockets, but at least he was disarmed and his attention had been temporarily distracted. Bellowing with rage and bewilderment, he took off across the pasture.

Having grumbled about my fee, which, considering the fact that I had risked my life, did not seem to me to be excessive, the owner began to tell me about his troubles. "I pray all the time, too," he said with a long face, "but it don't do a damned bit of good."

I countered by citing an increase in the price of drugs to be bought, and my client brightened. "Just a minute, Doc," he said. "I've got the very thing for you. Came in today's mail." He disappeared inside the house and emerged with a flyer advertisement for a Rexall one-cent sale.

Some six weeks later I had occasion to drive past his place. All appeared to be harmony once more. The bull lay in the shade of the cottonwood peacefully chewing his cud, his indignity obviously forgotten. The mule, still girdled by his now somewhat soiled bandage, grazed safely in the same enclosure.

Sometimes we felt justified in employing drastic measures to try to save an animal or to relieve its suffering, and for all that such an attempt requires courage, it can be rewarding if the end is successful. One day a client called to say his cow had an ear of corn lodged in her esophagus and was choking. In theory, it is impossible to cut into an animal's esophagus without causing death; but there seemed no other chance and so we took the risk, with the owner's blessing. We made the incision, removed the corn, and sewed up the wound. Happily, the cow survived.

On a hectic evening in the Oklahoma Panhandle, I had occasion to wish for three hands. A call came in from a widowed mother of two boys who was trying her best to farm the place following the death of her husband. The boys had been topping kaffir, she told me, and one of the mules had fallen onto a stalk of kaffir stubble, puncturing his side. The wound was bleeding badly.

By the time I could reach the place darkness had set in. I instructed one of the boys to hold the lantern and the other the mule, while I made the examination. The animal was breathing hard, indicating a respiratory disturbance, probably a punctured lung, I reasoned, and he was, indeed, bleeding profusely. The youngsters were understandably scared and upset.

There was something about the wound that puzzled me. It looked far too deep to have been inflicted by a stubble, and the aperture through hide and flesh did not appear to conform in shape. Such a wound is difficult enough to treat in broad daylight; I had only the flickering light of a lantern with a dirty globe. And presently I did not have even that. For the boy holding the lantern had slumped to the earth in a dead faint.

Handing the lantern quickly to the second boy, I splashed water from the instrument can into the first boy's face, and turned back to my job. "Crash" went the lantern a second time, as number two boy hit the dust.

Having brought him around by the same method, I sent the

pair to the house, and was left holding both mule and lantern while I finished sewing up the wound.

On the following day, the elder of the two boys came into the office to say that the mule had died. "We lied to you, Doctor," he confessed with an ashen face. Actually, the boys had been topping the kaffir with butcher knives, and when the mule crowded the untopped row to eat, the hotheaded younger brother, in a fit of anger, had jabbed the animal with his topping knife.

Medical doctors always complain that babies have a proclivity for arriving between sunset and sunrise. We discovered that the most troublesome calves are apt to do likewise, and that they also have a penchant for trying to be born in the foulest kind of weather. One bitterly cold night in Nebraska I was called out of bed by an apologetic client. "I've got a sick cow, Doc," he said. "I hate to bother you but I'm afraid if her calf's not pulled she'll be dead by morning."

Snow had fallen all through the day and was deep and drifted. The client's house stood a half-mile or so back from the road, his driveway bordered on either side by the kind of fence that promotes drifting. "You'd better not try the driveway," he told me. "Just turn into the alfalfa field down the road and follow the wagon track. We hauled hay out there today and the tracks will still show."

I got Dean out of bed, loaded my calf-pulling rig into the Jeep, and we set out. We made it to the farm without much difficulty, found the alfalfa field gate, and turned in. The light picked up the wagon track and we began to plough through the snow. The track skirted the trees and angled off toward a dim light we could see in the distance, but then turned back again to follow a crazy zigzag pattern, and then commenced to circle. Round and round we went, like children playing at fox and geese; but we hardly dared abandon the trail for fear of winding up in an irrigation ditch or bogging down in deep snow.

At long last we drew close to the looming barn, to find the anxious client waiting with his lantern. He asked whether we had had any trouble.

"No trouble," I told him. "But you sure ran a crooked course with that hay wagon."

"Oh, pshaw," he said. "I forgot to tell you, Doc. We had a little runaway this afternoon and made quite a few circles before we could get the horses under control again."

Most of our clients, as I have said, were sensible men who

knew enough to call us when they were in trouble beyond their own ability and knowledge, men who recognized the fact that their business was farming and feeding and that ours was doctoring, and we appreciated this. When an animal falls sick a time element may well be involved, and it is profitable as well as humane to get professional help as soon as possible.

But we encountered those, too, who felt called upon to try their own methods before calling us. One night we received a call from a local physician who owned a cow but who "boarded" her with an unsavory character who passed himself off as an amateur animal doctor. Had it not been for the fact that I respected the owner and felt sorry for the cow, I would have been reluctant to respond. The caretaker watched with ill-concealed amusement as I put a stethoscope on the cow. The familiar sloshing sound was evident.

"Sounds to me like she's got some kind of hardware in her heart," I said. "I doubt whether she'll pull through." There was nothing I could do for her.

A day or two later I met the keeper on the street. "How's Dr. M's cow?" I asked.

"Just fine," he told me. "I treated her. There wasn't nothing wrong with her heart."

A few hours later I had a second call from the physician. "My cow died, Doctor," he said. "I wonder if you'd go out and post her to see what was wrong."

I drove out, taking a helper with me. As before, the keeper watched with obvious amusement. Again, he made no comment, even when we found a bicycle spoke thrust through the diaphragm directly into the animal's heart. Leaving him to bury the cow, we were loading up our equipment preparatory to departure when my helper asked curiously, "Why do you suppose he had that tire tape wrapped around the cow's tail, Doc?"

"Hey, I noticed that," I said, remembering. "Let's go back and have another look."

We found the surly keeper preparing to bury the animal, and inquired concerning the tape.

"That's where I made the incision," he said. "She had wolf-in-the-tail. That's what she died of instead of that bicycle spoke." He had split the tail to the bone for a quarter of its length, sprinkled the wound with salt and pepper, and bound the cut together tightly with tire tape.

The Lord only knows how any ailment had come by that name, but we heard of it in other instances, too. Sometimes the incision was sprinkled generously with arsenic, presumably in an effort to drive out the "wolf." Another peculiar "disease" we often heard about in the timber grass country of eastern Oklahoma went by the name of "hollow horn." Of course the horns of all old animals are hollow. The method of treatment seemed to be to drill at the base of the horn and to insert some kind of patent medication, probably harmless save to the farmer's pocketbook. If a cow stopped chewing her cud she was presented with a greasy dishrag on the theory that she needed something to exercise her gums and needed lubrication.

On one occasion I was called upon to treat a colicky horse, long after the owner's treatment had failed to bring about a cure. Asked concerning the stinking contents of the gallon can from which he had administered generous forced drafts to the suffering animal, he told me it was a colic formula that had served his pappy well for forty years—a thick infusion comprised of water and chicken droppings.

We encountered a peculiar (and too common) trouble in the stockyards with animals shipped in for feeding. Many of these came from small farms where they had run about outbuildings, and we learned to look, when a cow turned lame, for a ring in the hair above one hoof or about one toe. We found that a bit of baling wire or a bit of packing wire had cut off circulation. Or we found a rubber jar ring such as was used, then, with zinc screw-on caps to complete a seal in home canning. Discarded each time a jar was opened, these rubber rings (for those who remember the method) found their way into farm dump heaps where the cattle ranged. With plenty of open space, farmers were pretty careless about where they deposited home discards. These stretched rings worked their way around the animals' hooves and gradually became embedded in the flesh.

I also recall a beautiful Collie dog, brought in once, with symptoms of tetanus or lockjaw. At first we were inclined to consider strychnine poisoning, unfortunately a fairly common occurrence with dogs. If you approached the animal or waved a hand in front of his eyes he went into tetanic spasm.

Presently someone more observing than the rest noticed a peculiar ring in the hair encircling the dog's neck, and we discovered that an embedded wire had indeed created a wound host for tetanus. The dog eventually died, a victim of childish ignorance, or human carelessness.

Any veterinarian who works with large animals has many calls to treat a condition known in the profession as "hardware disease," brought about by the ingestion of nails, screws, bolts, wire. Baling wire on a farm is one of the worst offenders. We saw many cases of *traumatic pericarditis,* an infection of the cardiac lining of the heart, caused by the penetration of such objects. These accidents are especially common with the cow, whose reticulum lies up against her diaphragm. Unfortunately, as with the physician's cow, we could do little save to verify our suspicions by posting. If a nail or wire enters the heart sac and sets up an infection, the animal is usually a "goner."

In later years, metal detectors came into use and it was fairly common practice for a doctor to operate. Magnets have been used, but with only moderate success. Occasionally a magnet inserted through a stomach tube will pick up a bit of offending hardware, but not often. One skilled surgeon achieved results by removing a rib and inserting a magnet through the resultant aperture. We knew dairy herd owners who routinely used magnets as a supposed preventive. Small magnets, inserted in capsules, were administered orally. Theoretically, the hardware attached itself to the magnet and dropped into the reticulum, where, supposedly, it did no harm. Perhaps the practice saved a few animals. Certainly it must have lined the pockets of a few glib salesmen.

Once, I was called out to look at a cow that had bitten the end off a gas pipe. The pipe had been threaded through a tube by the owner for the administration of some kind of medication and the cow had simply bitten the hardware in two. All I could suggested was that he keep a close watch. Sure enough she eliminated the hardware by a natural process.

Hardware disease was of such common occurrence as to nearly always come under discussion at veterinarians' meetings. I recall a question and answer period when a young doctor arose to relate an experience in which, during treatment, a client's cow had swallowed the doctor's capsule gun. He concluded, "What would you have done, Dr. K.?"

The learned man replied, "I would have charged the owner of the cow for the lost instrument."

It always seemed to me that the drawback in metal detector diagnosis lay in the fact that whereas the instrument might detect the presence of metal it might well throw you off the real cause of the symptoms in the animal's illness. Almost any cow's stomach will disclose bits of solder, nails, wire, that might have no bearing. We always found it more satisfactory to diagnose by stethoscope. If the animal's heart gave off a "sloshing" sound, as though it were beating in a pail of water, we came to be reasonably sure of heart penetration of some kind.

As an experiment, a group of Wisconsin students, bleeding cows for a brucellosis test, applied detectors to a total of three hundred animals. Seventy percent revealed the presence of metals, although none had displayed any illness. Such a pinpoint diagnosis (known as a clinical finding) is difficult and untrustworthy in even human patients, who can tell you where it hurts.

A fairly common hardware offender, especially with dogs, was a fishhook embedded in a lip, where it could be seen, or in a stomach where it could not. We always tried to work the hook around to where we could cut off the barb. If it had lodged in the esophagus, as it did sometimes, we had a problem. In porcupine country, we received many calls to remove the little barbed quills from a dog's face. Because of the pain inflicted by many barbs and the necessity for the animal to hold still, we usually employed an anesthetic. As a result of having been wounded, I suppose, most dogs have an intense hatred of the species and yet can't or won't seem to learn to leave the animals alone.

One morning we had a call from a farmer asking us to stop by and look at a horse that declined to eat. The owner suspected an infected tooth. The wife insisted that the horse could not swallow. Having inserted a speculum in the horse's mouth, I found nothing amiss with the teeth. But, feeling about at the base of the tongue, I encountered a sharp object: a sewing needle.

Here and now, I would like to pay my respects and express my gratitude to the inventor of the speculum, a device used to hold an animal's mouth open. Old time veterinarians employed the simple expedient of crowding the animal's tongue with a fist, on the theory that if he bit he crunched down on his own tongue—a good show, perhaps, but also a prime way to lose a finger.

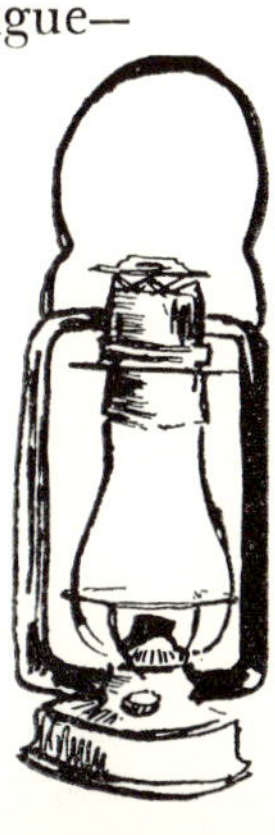

HORSE DOCTOR

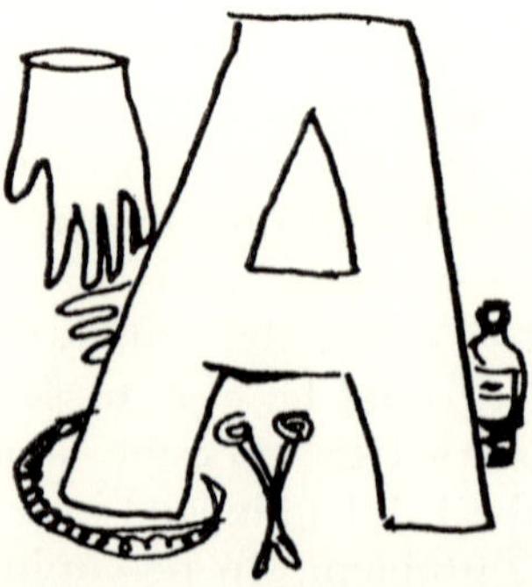

As children, we were always fascinated by stories about Dad's English brother, John Price, who had served as coachman and groom as well as veterinarian of sorts to a high-ranking family in Britain and then in Italy. Uncle John, whom we never met, had died at an early age of "quick consumption," ostensibly as a result of exposure during long evenings of sitting outside with his team and carriage to wait for his employers. As the only nephew with feet sufficiently small to crowd into them, I became the recipient of Uncle John's coachman's boots, which I wore proudly, and somewhat painfully, until they fell apart.

A second memento from Uncle John, which came to me late and which I prize highly, is a beautifully designed and lavishly illustrated volume entitled *Modern Practical Farriery*. Compiled by "W. J. Miles, M.R.C. U.S.L.," the book is "a complete guide to all that relates to the horse, its history, variety and uses . . . breaking, training, feeding, stabling and grooming . . . forming a complete system of the veterinary art as at present practiced at the Royal Veterinary College, London." The publisher was William Mackenzie, London, Glasgow, Edinburgh. No date of publication is given; but inasmuch as the list of members of the Newmarket Jockey Club is dated 1874 in the final column, I have a notion the book may have come into print about that time. I am also reasonably sure that this tome plus personal experience made up the sum total of John Price's education for his job. His name appears on the flyleaf, with the date 1880. Presumably he was already a young man, then.

The stylized prose names equine ailments, details the anatomy of the horse, and lists the turf celebrities of the day, classifying them as "roadsters," "hunters," and "trotting cobs." Horse medicines include anise, caraway, cassia, asafoetida, opium, strong ale, marshmallows, peppermint water, antimony, ginger, and rhubarb. As a kind of appendix or afterthought, the author has included an essay (not by him) on the diseases and management of cattle, sheep, and swine. No mention is made of the lowly chicken or of any other fowl. Although names given to individual diseases are frequently meaningless, certain symptoms sound familiar. Panaceas are for the most part simple and elemental: hydrochloric acid for "foot halt," effusion of pitcher plant for smallpox in sheep, and, for a variety of ailments, carbolic acid, lard, pitch, beeswax, quinine, chalk, and brandy. Udders of ewes were rubbed with camphor, goose grease, or spirits of wine.

Even as late as my own matriculation in veterinary school, when the horse was already on the decline as a draft animal, the sliding scale of importance placed the horse at the head of the list as patient, followed by cattle, sheep, hogs, and poultry, in that order. The "small animal," such as the dog and cat, was virtually ignored by most plains states professors of veterinary medicine. For sufficient reason, the first veterinarians were known as "horse doctors." Now the phrase has a kind of derogatory connotation.

During my childhood on the farm, stock owners had their own favorite remedies, most of them handed down. I came to see later that some of these made sense. The only times Dad called in a veterinarian were on those rare occasions when Old Bud the buggy horse became indisposed. Bud was a cherished member of the family and he also had a colorful history. Ridden by a neighbor of Dad in the "Osage Nation" (Indian Territory, now Oklahoma), the horse had made the Run at the opening of the Cherokee Strip. That his rider had failed to secure a claim was in no wise Bud's fault. All of the good land, the borrower explained, was already in the hands of Sooners who had jumped the gun. But Dad held to the theory that the wild young rider just may have lost sight of the purpose of the run in the excitement of the race and neglected to get down off his mount to drive stakes.

As I look back to those times, it occurs to me that barbed

wire was public enemy number one so far as the farm horse was concerned and that rusty nails ran a close second. Faced with barbed wire cuts during my own practice, I came to the conclusion that horses and barbed wire were never meant for the same era. Sometimes the animals were left with crippling cuts. Most of the injuries sustained around farms that kept horses were due to man's carelessness. I recall one lovely horse that took a bad foot wound when he stepped on a tines-up garden rake.

For barbed wire cuts as for other accidents and diseases, we used the simple medicaments kept on hand. Turpentine represented first aid for animals and for children and served as paint thinner as well. To keep wounds soft, we used "black oil." We applied Vicks Gall Cure to sore shoulders. For assorted cuts, sprains, and excoriations, we employed salves, ointments, and liniments obtained from the Watkins, Baker, or Rawleigh men, hucksters who traveled about the country by horse and buggy. We cured some animals. We lost some. A few survived, I suspect, in spite of our ministrations.

Often these itinerants arrived at mealtime. They were always fed. Occasionally we put one up, along with his horse, for an overnight. If he reimbursed us at all, he paid us in merchandise. Hospitality to a stranger was the rule, not the exception. I recall one plump, pious peddler who came on a Sunday morning (not to huckster surely) and threatened us with "the law" because he found us working in the fields on the Sabbath.

As a matter of economy and because he was fond of them, Dad took good care of his animals. Save during an emergency, the horses were turned out to pasture on a Sunday on the theory that a horse as much as a man needed a rest one day in seven. No heated animal was allowed cold water. Pads were used underneath collars. If a horse developed a gall he was taken immediately out of harness and the sore treated with lard and turpentine. We had occasional bouts of colic with horses as well as with children, and the former received about the same consideration and the same treatment as the latter. A sore teat on a cow was daubed with a camphor-smelling ointment kept on a shelf in the cowbarn. We rarely suffered any kind of an animal epidemic.

As a kid, I was always crazy about horses. I especially recall a kind of wonder horse we called Dick that seemed to sense

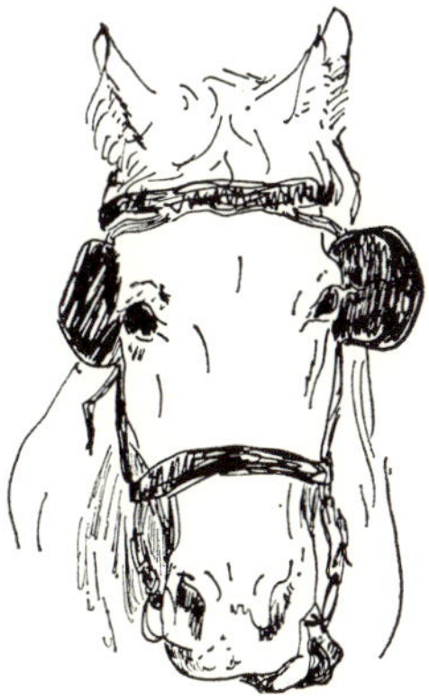

which way a cow was going to turn before she started. I felt a special rapport with Dick because I had brought him home as a pretty, iron-gray colt from the farm sale where Dad had bought him for thirty-five dollars. Never having had on a bridle or felt a bit between his teeth, Dick fought the metal as only a spirited colt would do. I had borrowed a saddle mare from a neighbor, John McGee, for the long trip down and back, and I tied the colt to the saddle horn.

We came along fairly well until we reached the Verdigris River, which was up about two feet from spring rain. The bridge across the river at that point had been condemned and it was necessary to ford the roily stream. Both mare and colt were afraid of the muddy, fast-flowing water. I finally persuaded the mare in, but the colt declined stubbornly to enter. When I got the colt under control, the mare balked. I suppose we were the better part of an hour negotiating the stream. By that time I think the colt trusted me a little.

Dad sold Dick, finally, to the cattle buyer Haz Reed, mentioned in an earlier chapter. When Reed came by one day to take away the small herd he had bought, we three boys were elected to go along with him the seven or eight miles to his stock pens, to help drive the cattle. Cattle were not hauled then, save by rail over long distances. To help with the drive, Reed had brought along an old black milk cow he professed to have trained as a bellwether. Once unloaded and started, the cow theoretically trotted ahead, and the herd followed.

Our cattle proved exceptions. When they reached the crossroads from which they could see the hill pastures over which they had gamboled and grazed during calfhood, they got a sudden homing instinct. Through the years we had learned to start any market animals off briskly and keep them scuttling until they got beyond any possible view of familiar territory. Otherwise no series of fences, however stout, would serve to contain them. The herd passed Reed's black bellwether in a cloud of dust and was a mile or more down the road before Reed and the cow caught up.

The cattle had settled down by then and Reed was in a talkative mood. As a boy of twelve he had witnessed the final raid of the Dalton boys in Coffeyville, where his father ran a general store. When the shooting started, he told us, a bystander burst into the store and asked for a gun and ammunition. Mr. Reed handed him a lever action Winchester and a box of shells and he ran out back to station himself behind a manure pile where the delivery horses were kept. Whenever one of the Dalton gang showed his head the sniper took aim and fired.

Contrary to popular belief, Reed told us, not all of the Dalton boys died that day. Four of them were killed, along with four of the citizens from the town. Emmett Dalton survived, was arrested, tried, sentenced, served his time, and then went into the real estate business in California—which may or may not prove he was rehabilitated.

As we neared the stock pens that day we came abreast of a squatter's shack with an old cow tied to a stake in front. There's something about a solitary bovine, loneliness I suppose, that motivates the animal to join any passing herd. This one pulled stake and came happily along. The squatter burst from his shack and accused us of stealing his cow.

"We can't cut her out now," Reed told him. "Just let her go. We'll bring her back when we get the others corralled."

The man seemed to acquiesce. But, a few moments later, having cut across a field, he leapt from behind a tree and made an effort to grab the cow's rope.

The entire herd took off like a covey of bobwhites. They went over and through a barbed wire fence into a cornfield in which tall corn stood among a jungle of cockleburs, morning glories, and high horse weeds. To make matters worse, the horses took fright and became all but unmanageable. By the time we got the horses under control and the cattle rounded up again, the field was ruined. Of course Reed had to pay for the damages. Ordinarily a good-natured man, he called the squatter all of the names in his repertoire, and made up a few.

Aware, that day, of Reed's admiration of my wonder mount, I wasn't above showing off a bit. A few days after the drive, he stopped by and asked Dad, casually, what he would take for Dick. "I just happen to know a fellow in Oklahoma who's looking for a good cutting horse and he might be interested."

"Well, he's a good horse," Dad said. "I reckon he ought to be worth a hundred and twenty-five." A hundred dollars in those days was a stiff price to pay for any saddle horse, stiff enough, I reckon Dad thought, to end the matter.

"This fellow won't go that high," Reed said.

"Well," Dad said, "I don't really want to sell him anyway."

"That's the way I had it figured," Reed said. He got out his checkbook and wrote out a check for one hundred and twenty-five dollars, and Dad had to let Dick go. I'm sure he hated to see the horse sold as much as I did. But at that time the check would have paid the taxes on the farm for a full year, and some dry, or wet, years our entire cash income from the crops didn't come to all that much. If it hadn't been for the eggs, chickens, butter, and cottage cheese ("Dutch cheese") Mother sold those years, pickings would have been slim sometimes. As children, we remained unaware that the fear of delinquency, the dread that we might lose the farm for lack of tax wherewithal, hung over our folks like a canopy of thunderclouds all the time we were growing up.

I could never call Dick my own, of course, but I did come by a good saddle horse a few years after the close of World War I. I had dropped out of school during the fall of 1917 to help on the farm during the absence of my brothers, Charles and Myron, away at war. But after the war ended I went back, and was graduated from Montgomery County High School with the class of 1921. During the summer and fall of 1921 and the spring and summer of 1922, I hauled gravel by horse and wagon for a county road building project. Wages of a dollar and a half a day plus a dollar for room and board were considered good for a man using a team other than his own and especially high for a kid without any experience at construction. I have thought since that spreading gravel was the best kind of incentive I could have had for seeking further education. We ate breakfast at four-thirty and supper at nine, and the work was pretty gruelling.

My brief career as a school teacher began in the fall of 1922. In those days, a high school education was considered sufficient for teaching rural children. My initial pedagogical effort took place in Foster District in the Sand Ridge country across the Verdigris River from home. The parents of my pupils, from grades one through eight, were mostly small truck farmers who eked out a living by producing watermelons and cantaloupes (called "mushmelons"), sweet potatoes, and sometimes peanuts, known as "goober peas."

This was pretty country, hills covered with scrub oak and persimmon, redbud, sycamore, hickory, and paw-paw trees, all of which colored beautifully in autumn. Oak leaves in shades of russet and scarlet remained on the trees throughout most winters, which were relatively mild. My salary was a whopping eighty dollars per month and transportation from home consisted of a heavy-footed combination buggy, saddle, and work horse named Logan. Logan could run all day without tiring, but he had two idiosyncrasies. He hated gravel roads and if you turned toward the county road off one of our soft farm access roads he was apt to whirl and take you back full-trot. Having once belonged to a rural mail carrier, he also drew up at each and every mailbox; so that, along routes heavily populated, we made slow progress.

It was during my second year at Foster with the munificent salary of one hundred dollars a month that I could afford a horse of my own. The horse's name was John, and he had a sad ending. I have often had occasion to wonder since if he could have been saved. I loaned him to a minister who had come to live on a place adjoining ours, to ride on Sunday to his church in Independence, a distance of about nine miles. Following the service, the parson chose to walk along with his girl friend to the home of a parishioner for a chicken dinner, leaving a young boy to ride the horse.

He had cautioned the boy not to allow the horse to go out of a walk, he assured me afterward; and I reckon the youngster heeded the admonition literally. Entering an intersection at full gallop, the pair collided with an oncoming automobile and was struck by a second car. Miraculously, the boy escaped injury. But, judging the animal to be mortally wounded, a policeman, hastily summoned, shot and killed the horse.

After nearly half a century, I can still see the dejected man of the cloth walking up the path to our back door late that evening, carrying saddle and bridle on his bent back.

Had I not already made up my mind to become a horse doctor if possible, a summer spent in Canada in 1924 would have clinched the resolution. Rural terms were seven months in length, then school closed in March, giving the teacher five months for a summer job and releasing the students in time to help with April gardening and corn planting. A recent law on the Kansas books decreed that a rural school must run eight months in order to partially close the gap between rural and nine-month urban institutions that were supposedly channeling better-equipped students into county high schools. But my school board, as well as many others, lacked sufficient funds to extend the term.

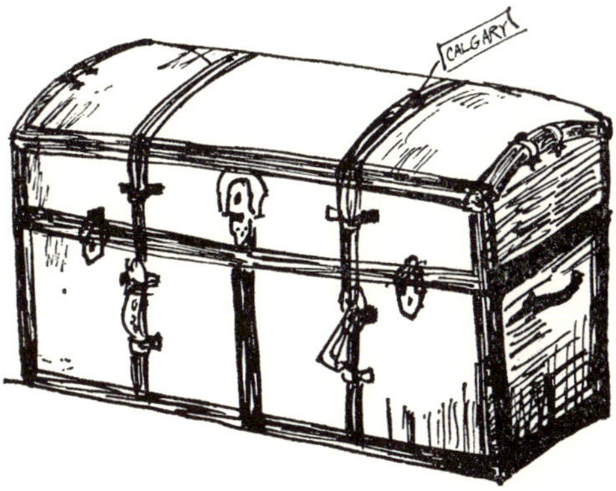

A few days after school closed in 1923 I had packed saddle and clothing into a trunk and set out for Nebraska to do farm work. The following summer, 1924, I spent on a wheat ranch in the vicinity of Calgary. Inasmuch as Edward the Sixth owned a ranch in the area, this was known as "Prince of Wales Country." Our Montgomery County neighbors, Jim and Jess Baker, had gone to the Province of Alberta when we children were young and had written back glowing letters about this rodeo capital of the Western Hemisphere. Show cattle went from Calgary to ports throughout the world and the area was noted world-wide for its blooded horses. In addition, the Dominion of Canada boasted good veterinary medical schools long before they were developed to a high degree in the United States. Indeed, the elderly practitioner whose practice I was to buy in Wisner, Nebraska, was a Canada-educated man.

I found that Calgary farming differed widely from any farming I had known. This was vast country and everything was big scale. A farm hand worked six or even eight head of horses. For planting, the animals were hitched three and three abreast, with two sets of lines controlling the outside pairs. For heavier work, such as sod-breaking, eight head were employed, four and four.

These beautiful animals were subjected to constant attack by botflies. To be sure, we had been bothered by these tormenting creatures in Kansas. But there the flies had deposited their nits on the animals' chests. Canadian flies, a different strain, laid their eggs inside the horses' nostrils, driving the animals half out of their senses. A second hazard with which we had to contend were badger holes into which the animals might step. As a result of some such accident, one horse assigned to me was so afraid of a badger hole that he would shy at the sight of one, crowding the entire team and making a botch in the plowing.

We worked six days a week. One-third of the land was kept under summer fallow, but it had to be constantly cultivated in order to be kept free of weeds. On Sunday I was at liberty to ride, and in that land of horses there seemed always one available for my use. We rode bucking horses "surcingle," without benefit of saddle. Sometimes I accompanied the family with whom I lived on excursions to pick Saskatoon berries, known as service berries in the States.

The vicinity of Calgary was rodeo-minded and there was much talk of riding and roping. There, rodeo riders were real ranch hands, not show people riding on mounts not their own. Rodeos drew riders from all the nearby ranches, and rivalry waxed lively between and among the cowboys. Flared wagons for hauling grain were called tanks. Towns being some distance apart, wheat had sometimes to be hauled for as much as thirty miles. For these hauls, six horses were hitched to a wagon, two and two and two. Good horse breeding was a matter of pride and organization. The Clydesdale stud used in our vicinity was brought around by his owner, and if we chanced to be at work in the field when he arrived we were obliged to unhitch and unharness the mare to be visited.

In the interest of keeping quality high, breeding fees were subsidized by the government. The Dominion paid one-third of the twenty-one dollar fee, the Province paid one-third, and the owner of the mare paid the remainder. This plan literally ran scrub breeding out of the business. Some owners had sixty, seventy, or even eighty brood mares, which, theoretically, might produce as many as thirty stud colts. From these, a provincial government committee was entitled to select the top three. The rest must be castrated.

In the fall of 1924 I went back to work as a teacher, in Cedar Bluff District near Coffeyville, at a salary of one hundred and twenty dollars per month. Having added architecture to my repertoire the following year, I was paid one hundred and twenty-five dollars. Desiring a new schoolhouse with very special specifications, the board asked me to plan the structure as a one-room, one-teacher school but with the upper four grades somehow separated from the lower four. The result was one large room, L-shape, the primary grades seated in one wing, the upper grades in the other, the teacher at such an angle as to, supposedly, keep one eye on each compartment, a good exercise for astigmatism.

On the way home from Canada in the fall of 1924, I had stopped off in Nebraska to marry Hazel Spangler, a sister-in-law to Harry Carrol for whom I had worked the previous year. We set up housekeeping in a small house in a grove of jackoaks in Sandy Ridge country and taught adjoining schools.

My own teaching career ended in the spring of 1926. I was twenty-four years of age. If I were to become a veterinarian, it was high time I started. Hazel was willing to help out with her teacher's salary. My first year of matriculation was at Independence Junior College in Montgomery County, where I had finished high school. In the fall of 1927 I entered Kansas State Agricultural College in Manhattan.

COW COLLEGES

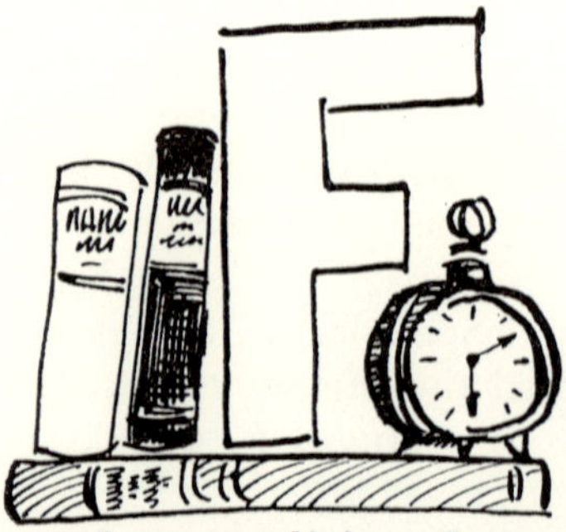

FREQUENTLY, these days, I find occasion to wonder whether I could gain admission to a contemporary school of veterinary medicine. In my time we entered veterinary college as freshmen fresh out of high school and had only to present our high school transcripts (which need not necessarily show a high average) and to express a desire to become veterinarians. The year I entered Kansas State the number of applicants was small. I doubt very much whether any were rejected. A few may have dropped out during the four years of my matriculation; we may have picked up one or two. My graduating class, in 1931, consisted of fourteen.

At that time the entire United States boasted no more than eleven schools of veterinary medicine. The number since has increased to eighteen or so, which still seems a very small number. In none of these, I am told, are there sufficient facilities to care for the number of students who wish to enter. One veterinary school, a year or so ago, accepted only fifty of the five hundred who had finished their preliminaries and applied. These fifty were top students, with a high grade average. Surely many of the others would have made good veterinarians. It seems to me that such criteria for testing may well leave out something to be desired. In a survey made recently by *Time* magazine, it was discovered that the relationship between course grades in most professional schools and occupational success in performance is in fact very low, often approaching zero.

Although we had much excellent instruction from some fine men, I had occasion sometimes as an early practitioner to regret certain practical gaps in our learning. It occurs to me that we had a good deal of useless theory crammed into our heads, or attempted. Of course, I could well be wrong. We did boast both in-patient and ambulatory clinics, and these were good. For the latter, we made calls when requested, usually on the coat tails of a professor, to look at some ailing animal or herd. For our service, if we performed any, the college received a nominal fee. Sometimes the referral was made by a practicing veterinarian, stumped, we liked to think, or faced with some ailment (such as fistulous withers) that he did not wish to handle. We encountered diseases on these calls that we would not see in years of practice and we saw too few diseases we were bound to be called upon to treat often as practitioners.

At times we received unusual animals as in-patients and I suppose we learned something from these. But who besides a zoo or menagerie doctor is called upon to administer to a wolf, a lion, a bobcat, or a monkey? I did learn one lesson concerning the latter species. Forgetting that he was more nearly *Homo sapiens* than *Felis domestica,* I grasped the skin at the back of his neck in a mistaken approach. With a quick twist he had me nailed with a Methodist grip on my working hand.

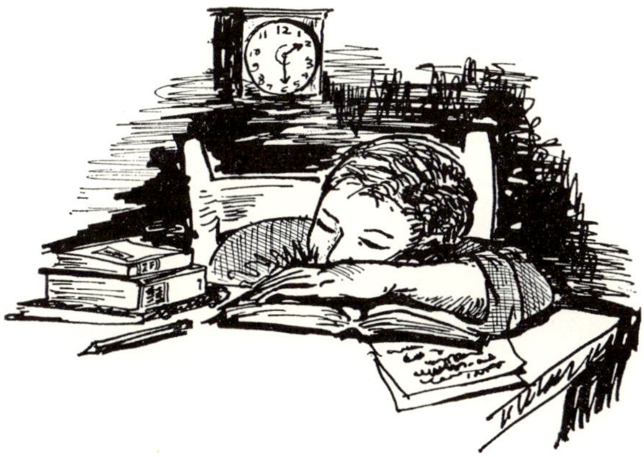

Times have changed for a veterinary graduate as well as for a practicing veterinarian, and I am not at all sure what my decision would be if I were among the former today. As large animal work has shrunk appreciably for the latter, many graduates I am told are being forced into such work as food inspection. This seems to be a waste of time and money spent both individually and by educational institutions for training. A groundwork of pathology and sanitation would probably suffice for this, certainly something less than the six years or so required to turn out a doctor of veterinary medicine.

Currently, some corporations devoted to the raising of livestock hire a "contract" veterinarian who agrees to care for a herd, to vaccinate, dehorn, castrate, and to treat at so much a head such ailments as may arise. I suppose such a contract would represent security of a sort; but it occurs to me, too, that the arrangement might well embrace some of the problems encountered in the human Medicare program. The veterinarian would be on call for the slightest digestive upset, with little time or energy left over for any other practice.

At the time of my own graduation, a veterinary student could finish college and obtain a degree to practice in four years time. As practitioners, we encountered veterinarians who had been educated on shorter order in private schools and some of these were very good. The Kansas City Veterinary College, absorbed later by Kansas State Agricultural College School of Veterinary Medicine, was one of the best. There, a full-fledged veterinarian could be turned out after three years of concentrated study, and a high school education was not a requirement for entrance. Too, certain smaller schools offered specialties that could be learned in a few months. I recall especially the Graham Breeding College and a school that taught a crash course in the rudiments of horse dentistry.

As a practitioner I found reason, often, to be grateful to various of my instructors for their efforts to instill a little good common sense along with technology. I have especial reason to remember Dr. E. J. Frick who taught us much that was extracurricular, not only about animals but about handling a certain kind of client. A diplomatic man, Dr. Frick could still be as tough as the situation demanded. I remember a call we received one day at the ambulatory clinic to go out and look at a herd of sick horses. The owner proved to be one of those individuals who had, or pretended to have, a contempt for academic learning and for those who were involved in such.

For all he had not hesitated to take advantage of any low-cost help or advice Dr. Frick had to offer, he appeared to want us to know that he looked upon us as a bunch of impractical greenhorns. Upon our arrival he pointed to the animals, some distance away across a creek, and launched into a dissertation concerning their symptoms. He then said with an unmistakable smirk, "Now you tell me what's wrong if you can Doctor."

As students, we would have been cowed I expect, but he had chosen the wrong professor to intimidate. "Look, Mr. ______," Dr. Frick said quietly, "we're *veterinarians,* not magicians. If you want us to look at your horses get some halters on them and get them over here."

Mr. ______ complied.

One of Dr. Frick's anathemas was the livestock owner who boasted about bloodlines. "Look at the *animal,* not at his pedigree," he told us over and over. A man who boasted of having bought a pup out of a five-hundred-dollar dog, he pointed out, might well prove nothing more than the fact that the pup's sire had cost too much. "Whenever the price of a purebred cow or sow reaches twice her market value as steak or sausage," he advised us, "she's probably reached her maximum worth. People are inclined to put too much stock in a piece of ancestral paper."

I was to recall his words many times during my years of sales barn inspection, when I saw animals bid up to exorbitant figures simply because of their illustrious lineage.

Occasionally an embarrassing happening occurred, even to the careful Dr. Frick. But these, too, were not without their peculiar instruction. Our entourage was called out one day to look at an injured steer on a large stock farm belonging to Dan Casement, who owned some three thousand acres of grassland in the Flint Hills north of Manhattan. When he had sized up the situation, Dr. Frick concluded that a subcutaneous dose of camphorated oil as a heart and nerve stimulant was in order, and this was administered. An account of the resultant aftermath was later related by Casement at a veterinary meeting where he served as a speaker.

Having decided that the injured steer stood little chance of a healthy survival because of a broken leg, the owner called in a butcher to slaughter the animal, and some of the meat wound up in a local market. On the following evening, Casement's perusal of the daily paper was interrupted by the ringing of the telephone. An irate female voice informed him that a certain Ladies' Aid Society had purchased a large roast for a church supper. The cooked meat had a "bad taste." The ladies had traced the product to the Casement ranch.

Casement put in a call to Dr. Frick and the two men headed for the church in an effort at appeasement. Frick sliced off a morsel of the beef, chewed it thoughtfully, and pronounced it all right. Reckoning that their own reputation as well as that of the ranch was at stake, Casement did likewise.

"I would as soon have taken a drink from the camphor bottle," he told us. "The ladies must have thought our taste buds had somehow deteriorated. The upshot was that we settled the matter by driving into town and purchasing sufficient hamburger to feed the multitude."

For the benefit of any novice who might administer camphor to an ailing meat animal, the lesson is obvious. There is nothing wrong with camphorated oil as a medication. But it should definitely not be given shortly prior to slaughter for market.

I like to remember that I worked for Dan Casement one summer at his Flint Hills ranch, putting in about four full days a week in the saddle and changing horses at noon. A Princeton graduate, as was his father before him and his son Jack after him, Casement ran for president of the United States on some obscure ticket in the year 1936. When he held a dispersion sale of quarter horses in 1954, I went down and bought two colts. Both made fine stock horses. A worthwhile article in the September 1971 issue of *Quarter Horse Journal,* authored by Benton Watson, pertained to Jack Casement and his work.

Probably the best turn Dr. Frick did for us was to teach us to take care of ourselves. Veterinary medicine even more than human medicine can be a hazardous occupation. One of the first requirements we made of the youngsters who helped us from time to time was that they learn how to properly tie a cow or horse prior to treatment. A primary precaution: Never have the knot of the rope near the snubbing post. You can always find a post around a barn or corral where you can make a half hitch. If you ever suffer a broken leg or choke an animal to death you will have paid dearly for having neglected this simple precaution.

Another professor I remember well was a Dr. Ibsen who taught genetics. A bit of a screwball, we thought then, he was still one of the few geneticists I have known who made a genuine effort to determine through meticulous record keeping which animal characteristics were apt to be inherited. For as far back as I could remember I had heard about a famous trotting horse known as Hambletonian, a stallion with a reputation so well established that the name was given to a strain of American trotting horses. If someone had a good trotting horse when I was a boy he was apt to refer to the animal as a Hambletonian Ten. Having compiled a track record of Hambletonian's descendants, Dr. Ibsen pointed out the fact that all of Hambletonian's colts out-trotted their sire; which all but proved, he declared, that the mares he bred were even better trotters than was the great stallion himself.

For our course in anatomy we were privileged to have Dr. W. M. McCloud, an authority on local anesthesia. Assisted by Dr. Frank, who taught surgery, Dr. McCloud did experimental work on epidural anesthesia for horses and dogs, a spinal anesthesia in which the solution is injected underneath the dura or outermost covering of the spinal cord. Inasmuch as we made use of horses in the anatomy laboratory, it was easy to follow the course of the dyed anesthetic solution in dissection. Many times during practice I had occasion to profit by Dr. McCloud's teaching. For obvious reasons, epidural anesthesia is far easier and safer to administer than is spinal anesthesia in humans, in which the solution is injected directly into the canal. I am inclined to agree with the anatomists who say that in more ways than one man would be better off had he never chosen to arise to an upright position and walk on two legs.

Dr. McCloud and I happened to have a common birth date. Presented with a cake, once, to celebrate his own natal day, he brought it to anatomy class. I will never forget the look of distaste on the face of a visitor who entered the lab that day, to find teacher and students enjoying refreshments in the midst of a room full of dead horses in various stages of dissection and putrefaction. Even with the use of a formaldehyde preservative, the horses got pretty high after a while. Dr. McCloud suggested that we learn to chew tobacco, and this helped. Liberal arts students often insisted that you could identify a vet student anywhere by the tobacco juice on his chin. We were somewhat taken aback when a later anatomy professor, who detested tobacco in all forms, announced at his initial session, "There'll be no tobacco chewing in this class." Sometimes he stood beside us to watch our work (we thought deliberately) until we nearly drowned.

As remarked earlier, approximately ten years prior to my

entry into college and all through my boyhood, a horse was an important member of farm economy. But by the time I was graduated in 1931 he was on the decline as a draft animal. If you wanted to belittle a veterinarian you referred to him as a "horse doctor." Still, Dr. Dykstra, the head of the School of Veterinary Medicine at Kansas State told us that in his native Holland it was more or less degrading for a veterinarian to be called upon to doctor anything *except* a horse. Dr. Dykstra looked upon the animals with which we worked in a descending scale: horse, cow, sheep, hog, dog, and, finally, chicken. He even spoke in a somewhat belittling manner of doctoring cows.

In practice, we came to know a few veterinarians who were half offended when asked to look at a flock of chickens. Indeed, when poultry diseases were first included in the curriculum they were put into "general science," instead of in veterinary medicine. Perhaps this peculiar snobbishness was somehow communicable; I have known very few poultry specialists in the field. Sometimes it seems that the entire profession has pulled away from farm and product consumer. Once, for example, a good cooperative relationship existed between animal health and meat inspection. Now the two departments often appear more like rival industries in which the right hand rarely knows what the left is doing.

As a middle-aged practicing veterinarian, I saw both my son Dean and my son-in-law Mike go through the same veterinary school I had attended. This gave me an opportunity to observe the changes that had taken place and to view these changes in the light of seeming gaps. Although I could see that many helpful courses had been added to broaden the veterinarian's outlook, I couldn't see that they were given much more actual medicine than we were.

Because of smaller classes, I suppose we received more individual instruction and also more clinical experience. In the comparative anatomy lab, for example, we had a carcass for every two students, and the carcass was not that of a dog or a goat, but of a horse. It goes without saying that this would not be possible in the crowded quarters of today's colleges. With larger classes and less space, thirty or forty head of horses or even of cattle would create something of a problem in logistics.

Although I realize that this could not very well be a requirement for entry, the fact of having been raised on a farm would seem to me to be of inestimable help to both student and practitioner engaged in large animal work.

In some cases, it is the sideline or extracurricular schooling that comes in handy. After a time in practice, I came to feel especially grateful to my high school manual training teacher for the rudiments he taught us about putting things together. Barnyard surgery at its sanitary best leaves something to be desired, and so we found it expedient to make boxes for the various kinds of work we were called upon to do most often. Equipped with hinged lids and with hooks at the back, these containers could be hung on some fence or manger near where the work was to be done. We had a large obstetrics box containing such items as a waterproof frock, wash basin, soap, pig and calf pullers, uterine capsules, disinfectant solution. The cholera box had compartments for such as serum and syringes. We made an erysipelas box. And so on.

Having arrived back at the office from a call, our first task was to clean whichever box we had used and to stock it with fresh supplies ready to go again at a moment's notice. With everything at hand that might be needed, without having to rummage through a bag for something perhaps forgotten, we could work with greater speed and less risk to the patient. In a small animal hospital it is realtively easy to create a sterile atmosphere. With barnyard surroundings, this is sometimes impossible, especially if the patients are hogs, not inclined by disposition to lead a very sanitary life.

If I were to venture a seeming comparison between the schools of today and of yesterday, I would say that a greater emphasis appears to be put on the small animal, the pet. I realize that university laboratories are better equipped to handle these and that small animal work has become a larger and larger field. It is interesting to note in this connection that recent statistics show that of the twenty thousand, six hundred practicing veterinarians in the United States, two thousand are licensed in California, and that of these two thousand, only one hundred and sixty-six do large animal work. On the other hand, the state of Wyoming has (or had) no strictly small animal practitioners at all.

For all that farmers are generally fond of their pets, a farmer's dog (and usually his cats) are members of his work force. We took care of them when requested, as a favor to our clients, but I cannot say that I particularly liked the work. I do not at all mean to say that there is anything unprofessional about pet work. I have been genuinely fond of dogs and of horses (especially the latter), and even of milk cows and of hogs. I know that in many cases, notably among lonely people, pets fill a psychological need.

I do have occasion to wonder sometimes about the unscrupulous practitioner who tends to prey upon the owner's emotions, to establish profitable pet cemeteries, to sell dog and cat coffins and the like. I heard of one doctor who sold an owner on the idea that she must give her dog only distilled water (purchased from him of course) to dissolve the animal's kidney stones. I am as intrigued by the fancy setups of some of the small animal hospitals as I am by the amount and variety of pet foods in the supermarket and by their cost. It occurs to me that we have come a long way from the farm where the dog (for all he was loved by the family) earned his way by sleeping outside to bark at an intruder, and helped with the livestock. Although he lived on table scraps, I think he lived about as long and as happily for the most part as does his more pampered prototype.

I like to remember that my own first mentor in the field of veterinary medicine was a cheerful little man who carried on a kind of itinerant dehorning practice among the farmers and stock raisers in southeast Kansas during the first decade of the century. I am not sure, now, of the little surgeon's name. It occurs to me that we called him "Rowe." Because Rowe's dilapidated wagon had for some reason been shortened so that the front wheels barely cleared the rear wheels while turning, the vehicle had a peculiar humpbacked look.

This informal mode of transportation, which carried all of the accoutrements of the owner's trade, boasted no spring seat, only a crossboard upon which the little old man sat enthroned; and his horses wore no breechings, only a simple crupper. As noted earlier, breeching harness was in those days a luxury item not often afforded by ordinary folk.

Dad did not dehorn every year. Sometimes two crops of spring calves were allowed to accumulate before we sent for Rowe. Perhaps we did not send, more likely Rowe simply stopped by on his rounds as did the scissors grinders and the salesmen for Capper publications. His surgical equipment was uncomplicated, consisting mainly of four items, a wooden chute that he hauled about in his wagon, a sharp knife, a small saw, and a can of creosote dip. Upon arrival, he unloaded the portable chute (which had a better head holder than our own), set out the dip can, placed his instruments on a nearby barrel or box, and fell to work.

With the animal's head securely laced to the headboard, he carefully sawed the horn at a precise angle and length to retain a border of hair about the base. When the appendage collapsed, he laid the saw down, picked up the knife, and deftly severed the remaining skin. He was not without his concession to cleanliness. Between patients, he cleaned knife and saw in the solution of creosote and water. He worked deliberately and with a professional air that we all found impressive. When he had finished we helped him to load his chute and watched him start on the ten- or twelve-mile trip to his home near Cherryvale, jogging along in his old contraption and singing or whistling to himself, I supposed in satisfaction over the work accomplished.

A man without formal education, he did the work he had learned to do, and he did it well. He had never heard the phrases, "social security," "public welfare," "new deal," or "great society." He would not in all probability have understood heart transplants nor craft that could exceed the speed of sound. He would most certainly have declined to believe that man would someday set foot on the moon. But I think he was a contented man. I know he enjoyed the respect of his fellows.

I have since observed many demonstrations by so-called experts in the field of dehorning and I have read and heard many learned dissertations on the subject. My own technique, followed through years of practice, differed little from the simple method employed by Rowe. Rowe advised, and Dad concurred, that the patients be kept cool and quiet. If a calf became overheated from running there was far more danger from bleeding. The only two calves I remember our having lost as an aftermath of dehorning died for this reason.

Rowe has long since departed this planet; he was in his sixties when I was a stripling. I suppose you might say that by current standards he barely made "a living." But he lived on that which he made. Seeing some of the modern concept illustrations of the banished Lucifer and his imps as creatures devoid of horns, I sometimes entertain the whimsical notion that Rowe may still be happily at work in some celestial region.

NATURE'S POISON CUPBOARD

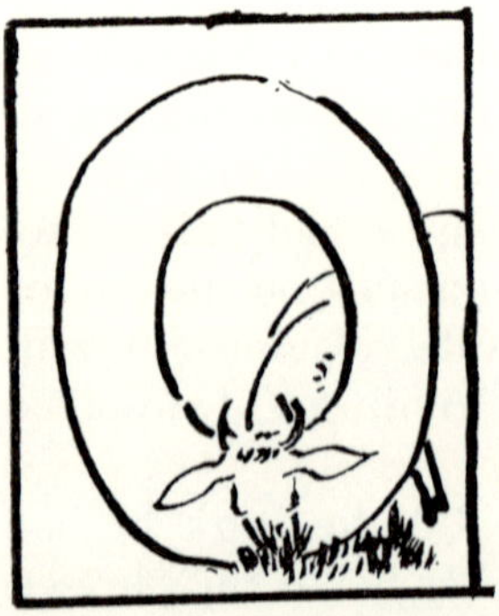

ONE OF THE MOST consistently painful and difficult assignments we confronted was the diagnosis of ailments brought on by the consumption of poison plants. A confusing factor in plant poisoning is that a plant may be perfectly harmless, even desirable forage, in one stage of growth and act as a deadly poison in another.

My own first knowledge that a common cocklebur could be lethal came when we received a call at the college clinic to a farm on the Kaw River to look at some dying hogs. The animals, it developed, had eaten cockleburs in the two-leaf or seedling stage. Another odd sort of accident, not to animals but to the farmer himself, occurred in the same area. The man had gone down to pick corn one morning when the dew was especially heavy. As he reached to break off the ears his hand repeatedly came in contact with dew-wet specimens of *Solanum nigrum,* the plant known as black nightshade. His pupils dilated and his eyesight began to fail. By the time he could reach the house he was temporarily, but totally, blind. Fortunately, he was rather quick to recover his sight and suffered no permanent damage.

A plant believed poisonous in all stages, even in hay, is arrowgrass *(Triglochin maritima),* a warm-season, grass-like perennial that grows near streams or in wet places. The adage that animals decline to eat that which is not good for them, save in times of scarcity, is only partially true. At home on the farm we had a bout or two with bloat (an ailment usually the end result of the ingestion of a legume) from green alfalfa, or from sweet clover. Once when we were laying corn by we lost a mare. To "lay corn by," is a term used for final machine cultivation, after which we boys moved in with hand hoes to chop out sunflowers, cockleburs, morning glories, and wild artichokes. The mare, a member of the cultivator team, bit the green corn as she moved along the row, and paid with her life for the treat.

Our method for treatment of bovine bloat was to stick the animal with a sharp knife "one hand's breadth forward and one hand's breadth down in front of the left side of the hip bone." Hopefully this incised the rumen where gas had accumulated. As a demonstration of the volatility of the gas, in the college ambulatory clinic we used to ignite the methane released when the trocar and cannula (the tube through which the trocar was inserted) entered the rumen.

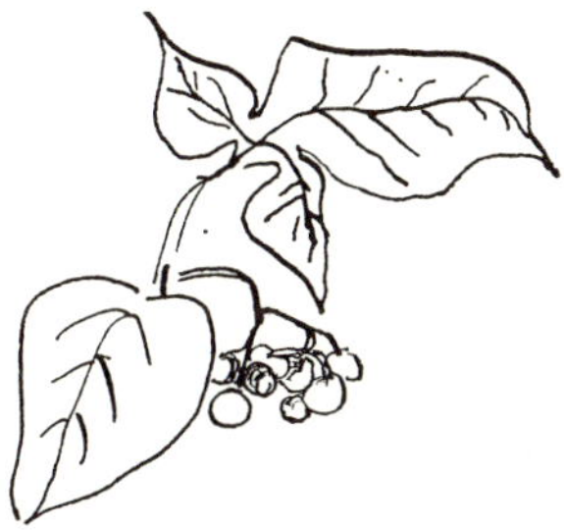

nightshade

All too frequently poisoning can be laid at the door of the owner of livestock or more likely an entire generation of owners. When desirable vegetation is eaten out down to bare earth, undesirable vegetation too often takes over. When good forage was killed in the central Nevada area by over-grazing, all that remained was cactus, too thorny for safe consumption, and plants unsafe because of their poisonous properties.

In some stages and in some areas, Russian Thistle constituted good forage, even though it had replaced a better. But like most desert plants thistle is filled with moisture in the green stage, causing a washy condition in cattle, known as "scours." During drouth and Dustbowl years, when we killed cattle that would otherwise have died of starvation, we killed closer where animals had been kept alive on Russian thistle. A cow that had eaten only thistle might be in fair flesh but die during the trip to the railroad yards or in the shipping car.

Loco weed, or woolly loco *(Astragalus mollissimus),* another legume, gave trouble in both Oklahoma and Nevada. A peculiar and insidious fact about loco is that it is habit-forming. Once an animal started eating the weed, she would scarcely touch anything else. Horses addicted to loco became wild, solitary, and uncoordinated, stepping high over low obstructions and shying at their own shadows. A strange symptom of loco poisoning in a horse is the lengthening of the tail. The tail of a horse hooked on loco will all but touch the earth sometimes.

One of the most interesting and also one of the most devastating problems we dealt with in Nevada was a disease called *molybdenosis* that came of an animal's having grazed over an area with a high concentration of molybdenum. Following a heavy dose of molybdenum an animal's body becomes deficient in copper, and anemia results. This condition was especially evident in the anemic appearance of the blood when we dehorned calves. As we drove along the road, we could see, even from a distance, when animals suffered from the disease, by the light yellow spots that marked their coats. The hides of black Angus turned mouse color.

Treatment was simple enough; we injected copper glycinate into the brisket, and sometimes saw near-miraculous benefits. We also advised adding copper to the diet. Logically enough, in sections of Wyoming where soil contained an excess of copper, molybdenum came into use as a supplement, or as an antidote. Where a proper combination of the two obtained in the earth, they appeared to balance each other.

One peculiar affliction we saw a good deal of was a kind of sunburn in hogs, especially in white or light-colored breeds, a hepatogenous photosensitization brought about by the ingestion of wild rye, buckwheat, St.-Johns'-wort, and other plants of the genus *Hypericum* that affect liver function. Most of these grow in wet places. St.-Johns'-wort, a fairly common weed, is listed as moderately poisonous but only to white or light-colored animals.

In Nebraska, once we underwent an odd experience with a *Polygonum* we called "smartweed," or, erroneously, "redroot." The owner of a herd of cows stopped in one morning to complain that the animals' teats were so sore that he could hardly manipulate them. Thinking that the cows might be afflicted with cowpox, an eruptive disease, I gave him an ointment we used for the purpose. The following day he called to ask me to come out.

The cows presented a startling appearance. Their hind parts, unprotected by hair, glowed red in patches that had a leathery texture. The teats looked, indeed, awful. When the owner, upon questioning, told me the animals had broken into a potato patch I asked to have a look at the area. Smartweed grew rampant.

We gave the animals injections of antihistamine and treated the patches locally. The condition cleared and teats healed, but the skin peeled off, leaving areas like ancient leather. Passing by the place days afterward, I saw strips hanging as dead bark hangs from a cedar bole. But, then, the new skin that appeared was as fine and as silky as that of a newborn calf.

Sometimes we saw the same kind of photosensitization in the white belt around Hampshire hogs. Strong sunlight does not penetrate dark skin or clothing. We saw so much skin cancer and other trouble in *humans* in sunny Nevada that it came to seem that the modern Nevada cowboy was in error when he turned his hat up at the sides instead of leaving the brim down all the way around, as had his earlier counterpart. My brother-in-law, Dan Furse, has a favorite theory, to the effect that cowboys in New Mexico turn their hats up on the sides so that more can sit side by side in a pick-up truck.

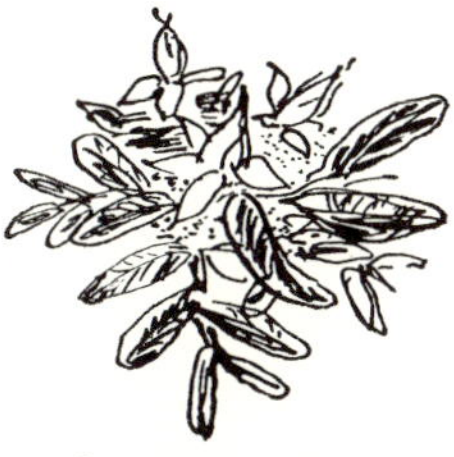

St. Johnswort

I recall another poisonous plant that emerged in Kansas pastures when the grass shortened in the fall following a long dry summer. This was a hairy little croton, containing a cathartic oil that caused animals to scour. Dad referred to the condition, as I recall, as "dry murrain" or as "bloody murrain," a word also applied to Texas fever, to anthrax, or to hoof-and-mouth disease.

During our cattle buying junkets in Oklahoma we sometimes encountered an ailment referred to in our orders as "frozen foot," a condition caused by an ergot (a word familiar to human abortionists), a parasitic fungus that replaces some of the seeds in various cereal grains such as wild rye and brome. We had an interesting and enlightening observation of this fungus once during a trip to Sterling, Colorado, feed yards.

As I was walking down the alley between the pens with a yard hand, I began to notice aborted calves. Sometimes pregnant heifers in feed yards are deliberately aborted, and so I took this to be the case and asked the hand whether he had given the animals stilbestrol.

"We've got something better than that," he told me. "And cheaper. I just give them a big feed of milo."

"Milo won't abort an animal."

"Works every time," he insisted stoutly.

It occurred to me suddenly that the milo he was feeding was probably half ergot!

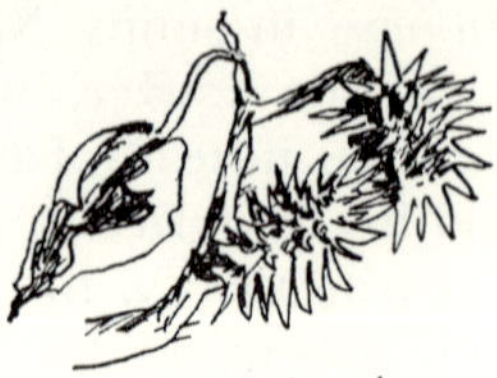

Cocklebur

Every now and again we came across a case of salt poisoning in hogs, especially among owners who held to the old wives belief that when you changed feed you must add salt in order to help the animals adjust to the change. A salt poisoned hog lies on his side and thrashes with his feet as though with a bellyache. Post a hog that has died of salt poisoning and you find a highly inflamed intestine.

I think I can say without reservation that if there is one disease or epidemic a veterinarian dreads more than another it is cholera. At least this was the case with me. When I received a call one day (in Nebraska) from a client whose hogs I had vaccinated against the disease, I lost no time in getting there.

The hogs were in bad shape all right, but symptoms pointed, rather, to some kind of plant poisoning. Knowing that he had been bothered from time to time by nightshade *(Solanum),* I asked whether he had checked this out. He had found some nightshade earlier that spring, he told me, but he had sent his son and the hired hand to chop it down and he was sure they had followed instructions.

The pair had chopped the plant down, we discovered. But they had neglected to burn the residue. We found *Solanum* "hay" all over the lot. Perhaps it tasted even better in the cured stage and it may well have been even more lethal in a dried condition. Our best efforts to save the animals that had fallen ill were largely futile. He lost a total of fifteen hogs to the poison.

Turned out after being confined all winter on a grain diet, a hog will go "hog wild" for a taste of green. We used to warn owners facetiously to paint their John Deere tractors any color but green if winter-bound hogs were to have access to the implements. When such a newly released herd fell sick one morning we were called out.

We found nothing growing in the feedyard itself that might cause harm. But outside and in close proximity to the fence grew specimens of hemlock, as Socrates well knew, one of the deadliest poisons known to man. A strong east wind, we reasoned, had blown the plants against the fence. The hogs had eaten every available leaf and had rooted underneath the fence in search of more. Sixteen of the animals died on the spot.

"But why did they eat it?" the unfortunate owner asked again and again, as though an answer to that mystery might serve as a resurrector. All we could do was to sympathize and to point to the ravenous greens hunger of animals too long restricted to a dry fare.

A second *Solanum,* wild ground cherry, also gave trouble at times. Not quite so toxic as deadly nightshade, a little of this herb will still suffice in some stages of growth. As stated earlier, a peculiar fact about some of these poisons is that, undamaged, they make good forage. A case in point is Sudan grass, rather widely planted in Nebraska as a food. Damaged, the grass generates a poison. But, then, when the same plant is dried, the poison factor is volatilized and hay can be used with perfect safety.

Prussic, or hydrocyanic, acid poisoning comes usually of animals having eaten certain of the sorghums, such as one of the canes, damaged by dry weather, trampling, or frost. Following such abuse, the chemical composition of the plant undergoes an alteration. Too frequently the victims were dead by the time we arrived on the scene.

An instance of the way in which a plant may change from nontoxic to toxic overnight happened in Oklahoma. Shortly after harvest time, a farmer called to report four dead milk cows in his herd. He had been feeding nothing special, he assured me. He had been turning the animals out on grain stubble in the afternoons but he had searched the field carefully before doing so to make sure that nothing grew there that might bring them harm.

Indeed, he was turning the remaining animals onto the stubble when I arrived. From where we stood, I could see that Johnson grass, a good forage, had come up thick following the harvest of grain. The animals surged through the gate and scattered. As we watched, one, two, three, and then a fourth went down. As we ran to drive them back out of the field, one old cow fell across a tree root. I stuck a needle into her jugular vein.

Her blood was the color of chocolate syrup, a telltale indication that some poison had formed a stable compound with the hemoglobin, depriving her tissues of oxygen. The Johnson grass!

At one side of a range of mountains south of the town of Ely, Nevada, a group of Mormons ran cattle over an area known as Horse Camp. The drive to pasture on this range led over the mountains forty miles south of Ely, where nothing much in the way of forage grew. So that by the time the animals began the descent down the slopes to Lund and came upon the plant named halogeton, they were ravenous. *Halogeton glomeratus,* easily recognized in its earlier stages, is sometimes mistaken in maturity for Russian Thistle. Many animals sickened, and some died, from gorging on this rank specimen.

Seeds of halogeton generally lie dormant until the earth is somehow disturbed. On one occasion when a crew bulldozed a new road grade the plants sprang up like Jason's army. Salt-deprived animals have a special penchant for halogeton because of the salty taste. For this reason, we advised ranchers to make plenty of salt available, well away from these heavy yields that might attract.

Greasewood gave us some anxious times, though with this plant the lethal damage is more mechanical than toxic. Covered with spines, the plant, once ingested, may lie in the rumen and damage the walls of that organ so severely as to cause death. Some animals fall victim to plenty. Given a surplus of good forage, they die of overeating, just as some humans (indirectly) do. Yet who would consider a New York cut a lethal product?

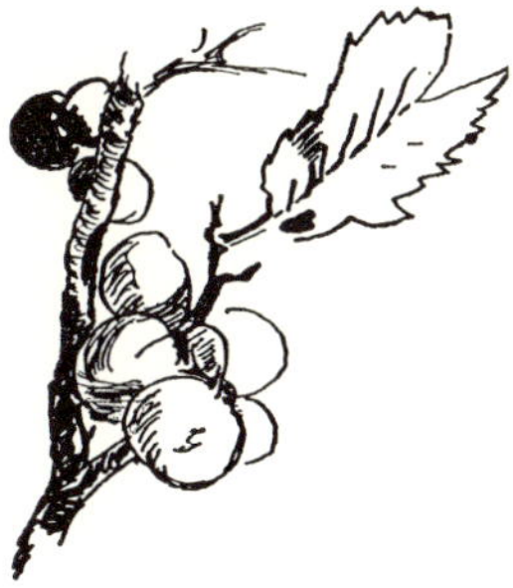

Wild plums

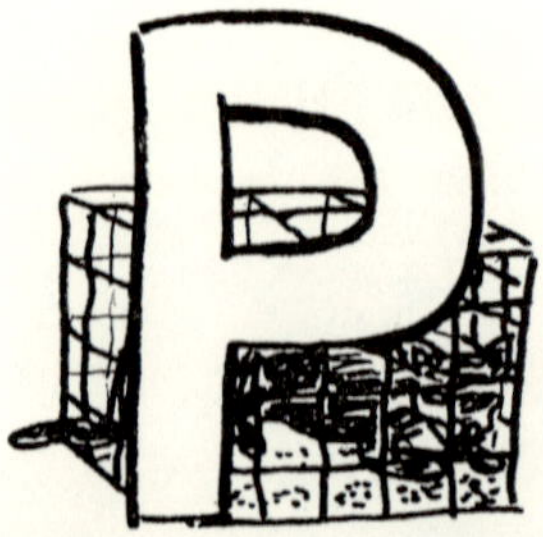

PROBABLY the most frightening of all the diseases a veterinarian meets in his tour of duty is the dread condition known as rabies. The only way in which the ailment can possibly be positively diagnosed is by waiting until the animal dies and sending the head into a good dependable laboratory for analysis. Yet, despite repeated warnings, people panic and kill the suspect and so destroy the evidence.

The first rabid animal I was called upon to treat was in Oklahoma. While testing cattle near Stillwell I received a call from the county agent to go to a certain farm and have a look at a cow acting suspiciously. I found the animal, a little Jersey, a pet of the family, tethered by a heavy rope to a small peach tree. Ordinarily mild-mannered, the owner told me, she had suddenly become unexplainably belligerent. If a pebble were tossed in her direction, she charged the object with seeming anger. Even when a butterfly approached she ran at the insect until she reached the end of her tether. She kept up a constant drooling and bawling, almost sure symptoms of rabies in cattle.

When she had first fallen ill, the owner explained, he had called in a "lay veterinarian" of his acquaintance. Thinking she might be suffering from an obstruction, this good Samaritan had thrust his hand down her throat, but had found nothing. And so the farmer had gone ahead and milked the cow. His children had drunk the product as usual.

This latter fact filled me with uneasiness. I could see that the animal suffered from some disturbance of the central nervous system and I didn't at all like the symptoms. In language as strong as I could make it, I instructed the owner to stay clear of the cow, to keep the children and all livestock at a distance, and to see that the animal remained securely tied. I would stop in on the following day, I told him.

By the next morning I could see that her condition had worsened, that she suffered from some paralysis. Believing that death was imminent, I told the owner that he must in this event send the head to the state laboratory without delay. I was uncertain as to what the drinking of her milk by the children might mean in case my suspicions were confirmed, but I could not help thinking about the fact that they had done so.

To my surprise, the farmer objected. To ice and ship the head would cost a great deal he told me. His friend had not mentioned rabies. She showed no signs of having been bitten and he had seen no stray dog around. In short, he doubted my diagnosis.

All of this talk got my dander up. I would remove the head free of charge, I told him. But it was his family, after all, that had possibly been exposed, and he was far better able than I to pay the shipping bill. After much argument, he contacted an uncle, who volunteered to meet the expense.

A wire came promptly from the state lab. The cow was, indeed, rabid. Pasteur treatment was to be sent immediately to be taken by all who might have been exposed. How many were there?

I consulted the local medical doctor, who concluded that the entire family had better be treated. How about the friend who had his hand down her throat?

"We'll just forget about him," the M.D. responded charitably. "That SOB's too ornery to come down with even rabies."

On the following day, one of the owner's neighbors called in great alarm to say that two of his cows were acting in a peculiar manner. Although he lived five or six miles from the first and there had been no contact between the animals, these also proved to be rabid. We feared an epidemic, but no other incidents occurred that I heard of, and the source of the infection remained a mystery that kept us uneasy for a long time.

A good while afterward, in another area, I was called upon to look at a cow with identical symptoms. This one had chased her owner to the top of a straw stack in a sweet clover patch, from which he had experienced some difficulty in escaping to call me.

"I don't know what's got into her," he said. "She's usually as gentle as a lamb. But this morning she'd fight a buzz saw."

My helper, a boy who roped well, told me he thought he could get a lasso on the animal. As we approached, warily, she got up, with obvious effort, swung her head from side to side in an ominous manner, as though to pinpoint our voices, and charged the spot where she thought us to be. At each attack, we retreated, and then moved forward in such a way as to try to remain out of focus.

During this maneuvering, the owner's son, who had been away and knew nothing of our problem, roared into the field in an open Jeep. The ensuing scene was like a Laurel and Hardy comedy. Ignoring our shouted warning, he stepped out of the car.

In a burst of speed that would have done credit to a racehorse, and with good aim, she charged the youngster, who ran for the Jeep, leapt behind the wheel and grabbed the gear shift lever. The knob came off in his hand, the cow hit the Jeep at a hind wheel, lifting the car so high off the ground that her intended victim spilled out the opposite side, and lit running.

When the cow fell, finally, exhausted, we got her roped and tied. This time we did not have long to wait for death. When she, too, proved rabid by laboratory test, we questioned the owner as well as the neighbors to see whether we could come at the source of the disease. We never did, really. We did learn, for what it was worth, that a number of dead skunks had been found in the area within the previous month. The skunk had been for some time suspect as a carrier, but we could only surmise in this case. Fearing that hogs or chickens might eat the animals and come down with some disease, farmers had systematically gathered and burned all the carcasses. Whatever the source, we heard of no recurrence. But, again, neither we nor the farmers in the area relaxed our vigil for a considerable period.

The coinage of the word "hydrophobia," a common name for the disease, came originally of the belief that a rabid animal possessed some peculiar fear of water. Later researchers concluded that the frantic reaction to the sight, the sound, or the smell of water came from the victim's insatiable thirst and of an inability to swallow due to a constriction of throat muscles. I have seen a rabid cow throw a tantrum at the mere sound of water being poured into a bucket, a distressing sight but an almost invariable symptom of the malady.

A more or less amusing incident to do with rabies occurred when I was still in college. As an upperclassman in veterinary medicine, I had been placed in charge of the clinic where we kept ailing animals brought in for observation. When Christmas time rolled around I went home for a few days, leaving a local boy to feed and care for the patients and to keep the place clean.

Upon my return, a day or two after the holiday, I saw that a new dog, a Collie, had been brought in during my absence and that his kennel bore a RABID label. We received a suspect every now and again. We could, of course, only wait until the animal died in order to confirm any diagnosis; but the kennels of such animals were always carefully labeled with a warning sign. On the following morning I was astonished to see that the RABID label had been transferred to a cage containing a coon hound, brought in for some ailment also not yet diagnosed. Puzzled, I rounded up the beginning student who served as janitor. "What goes on here?" I asked. "This sign was on the Collie's kennel yesterday."

"Is that where it was?" he ejaculated. "When I opened the door to sweep out last night the card blew off onto the floor. I didn't know where it belonged, so I just got to watching the dogs. I finally decided from the crazy way this coon hound acted that it belonged on his cage."

The boy proved right. The coon hound was rabid!

Once in Oklahoma when we thought we had a bad near-epidemic of rabies, the condition proved otherwise. One Sunday morning I had a call from the superintendent of the State Mental Hospital at Supply asking me to come down and have a look at some cows that seemed suddenly to have taken leave of their senses.

The animals looked as though they belonged in some kind of mental institution all right. Several had died, the superintendent told me. The survivors mostly sat about on their haunches like so many dogs, or assumed the weirdest kinds of postures. "It looks more like some kind of poisoning," I told the worried staff doctor. Neither of us thought, really, that the animals could be rabid, but we were both mystified, and with a public institution you don't dare take chances. We removed the head from one of the dead animals and drove into Oklahoma City to the laboratory. The test proved negative.

The answer? A maintenance crew painting one of the buildings had left the "empty" paint cans lying outside in the cow lot.

Having licked the cans clean of the last drop, the animals were sick, and dying, of lead poisoning.

That day proved memorable for another reason. While I set about posting the dead animals, the superintendent issued orders to the effect that certain of the patients were to dig holes in the dry ground to bury the remains. One fellow refused. He dropped his shovel and concealed himself behind a row of barrels.

Hastily summoned, a bevy of guards arrived on horseback armed with ropes, as though they meant to lasso the holdout. Whenever one of the guards approached, the now thoroughly aroused patient threw a barrel stave at the horse. The horses were in a panic from the flying staves and all was pandemonium.

Backed, finally, against a building, the patient threatened to throw a doorknob at one approaching guard, who, sensibly, came to a halt. The inmate was a husky fellow. Had he thrown the knob, with good aim, he might well have killed his pursuer. But that day I began to place a certain credence in the rumors that certain guards hired by this institution and by other minimum security places were sadistically inclined.

Not long afterward, a considerable scandal broke. Following some incident of insubordination, one such recalcitrant was actually roped by a guard and dragged to death behind the guard's horse. The guard was brought to trial. Several patients had witnessed the affair, but their testimony proved unacceptable because of commitment to a mental hospital.

Thanks to the lawyer for the prosecution, a stubborn injustice fighter, the case had a happier ending than most. Patiently screening the records of the witnessing inmates, he found one who had been railroaded into the institution by scheming relatives, a none too uncommon practice. Having proved beyond a doubt that the witness's testimony was acceptable, the attorney put him on the stand. The guard was found guilty.

As an aftermath of the trial this particular hospital and some other public institutions in the state came in for a thorough and much-needed investigation.

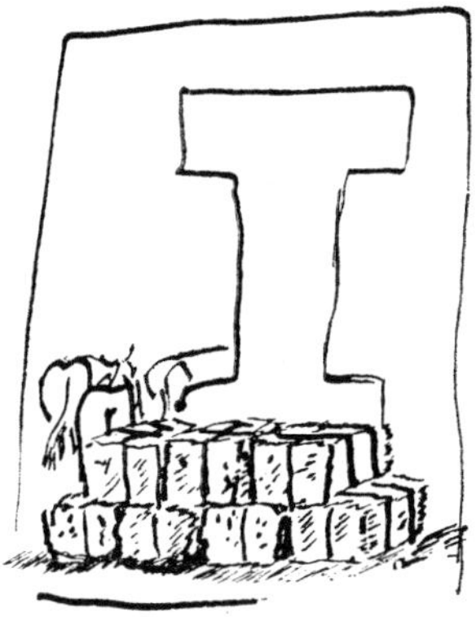

I DON'T KNOW how it is with other professions; but it always seemed to me that some of the most worthwhile values, as well as the most fun, to come out of veterinary meetings materialized in the hotel rooms set up for advertising purposes by serum and drug companies, which also, of course, furnished better whiskey than most of us could afford. You might well sit through some long-winded talk with tongue in cheek, afraid to speak out or to ask a question for fear of exposing your own ignorance, and then learn, upstairs, that most of your colleagues had done likewise.

I recall a talk concerned with the vein bleeding of hogs as a testing device. As anyone who has ever tried to get a needle into a hog's vein will agree the operation is usually one hell of a job. The speaker had made it all sound ridiculously simple. We were discussing the talk afterward, upstairs, most of us kibitzing, when one elderly practitioner translated the matter dryly into words.

"Well, gentlemen," he said, "I've attended veterinarians' meetings all my working life. And personally I've always found that hogs are a good deal easier to vein bleed on the speakers' platform than they are in the hog lot."

Mechanics in the field, he was saying, can no more be learned on the lecture platform than in the classroom. Each case is individual. How do you catch the animal? Where do you tie it? Where do you lay out your instruments to keep them as sterile as possible? And, last but by no means least, which way do you jump following an injection?

When spirits were lifted by lifted spirits, not a little bragging ensued, along with, I suspect, considerable exaggeration. When the talk turned to fees and economics of practice, once, one of a pair of brother veterinarians in practice together remarked modestly that the biggest business day he ever did brought in around one hundred dollars.

From a hidden cubicle came an astonished ejaculation, "That's news to me, brother John! Maybe you'd be so good as to tell me what the hell you did with my share."

As upperclassmen in college, we became pretty blasé sometimes when younger, less experienced students were out with us on an ambulatory case in the field. I reckon those of us who had been lucky enough to grow up on a farm were especially obnoxious. I remember a case involving a big mule and one of those situations that call for some ingenuity as well as know-how.

Tormented by his wound, the mule looked both mean and mad. Having nothing in the way of a twitch available, we made one from an old pickhandle by boring a hole and passing a rope through the aperture. A student held the twitch while the professor in charge examined the mule. Having come to the conclusion that the animal should have an anti-tetanus injection, the doctor assigned a younger student to give the shot.

The student (I'll call him George) approached the mule warily enough. But then, instead of the quick jab and fast getaway, he inserted the needle slowly. I don't know how George escaped the rebound. I was on the run by that time, as were most of the others, including the good professor. The sole casualty was a passing dog, struck by the flying pickhandle.

One of my favorite convention stories has to do with a load of Brahma bulls, flown to Brazil for breeding purposes. I suppose the tale has been told many times and that it has lost nothing in the telling. It is none the less purported to be true.

For the scheduled flight, the passenger cabin of a big freight plane had been fitted out with stalls, into which the animals were tied. All went well during the first leg of the journey. But then somewhere over Mexico, according to an eyewitness, one of the big animals managed somehow to slip his head out of the halter. Alarmed by the roar of the engine and his unfamiliar surroundings, he began to charge up and down the corridor. As the frightened attendant tried without success to get the bull back into his stall, and the plane rocked with the shifting weight, a white-faced captain appeared in the doorway to the cockpit.

"I can't keep this crate in the air," he shouted. "You'll have to *do* something!"

"Can't we land?"

"Impossible! We're over high mountains."

The bull charged the new voice. The other animals strained at their ropes and set up a bellowing. The plane lurched. The pilot hastily retreated.

With an ingenuity born of desperation, the attendant worked his way to the tail section, where he managed to unlatch and to push open a passenger door just as the bull turned and came toward him. The Brahma went through without a moment's hesitation and was lost in moments among the clouds. "Seeing as how the skies were raining Brahmas," the teller concluded, "I'll bet some siesta-taker down there threw away his half-empty mescal bottle."

Sometimes these stories took the form of confessions. None of us was immune to occasional goofs that seemed funny in retrospect. One of my own prize goofs had to do with milk fever, and I told the story to my dentist long afterward, when he was preparing one day to extract a molar for me. As he waited for the anesthetic to take effect, poking and prodding now and then with his instrument, we fell to discussing procaine, a novocaine synthetic.

"You don't dare hit a vein with this stuff," the dentist declared knowledgeably. "I learned that the hard way. Patient fell out of the chair as though he'd been hit with a poleaxe."

"Maybe not a human vein," I told him. "But I remember a cow once . . ."

Luckily for me, the incident occurred at the edge of a thicket, in dustbowl country. My patient was a little Jersey, suffering from milk fever, a too-common ailment in that area. Inasmuch as no satisfactory way had been devised to keep calcium gluconate in solution, I used calcium chloride, injecting the drug into a vein slowly in order to guard against heart shock.

For these injections, I had formed the habit of using and re-using two hundred and fifty-cc bottles, which we sterilized in the pressure cooker between fillings, marking the contents plainly on the stopper.

That day, I violated the first precept of medicine. I picked up the bottle without so much as a glance at the label and got procaine instead of calcium chloride. It was not until after I had injected eighty cc's of the stuff and withdrawn the needle that I saw to my horror what I had administered. Throwing bottle and cork quickly into the thicket, I grabbed the chloride bottle and injected one hundred and twenty cc's of that as a chaser.

The dentist asked, "What happened?"

"Well, I don't know what happened inside the cow," I told him. "I can say this, she got up and walked away as though she had never been sick a day in her life."

One of the most bizarrely dramatic stories to do with the profession was told to me by an older veterinarian, as a personal experience. Although I was never called upon to employ the tactic, we were told in college that one humane method of destroying a horse or mule that had to be done away with was to tie the animal securely, wire half a stick of dynamite to his halter, and light the fuse.

Called out to look at a mule that suffered from a bad case of glanders, this particular veterinarian had told the owner the case was hopeless and recommended that the animal be destroyed. "He said he would like me to do the job, but that he had no gun on the place. I asked him whether he had any dynamite. Well, yes, he had, he said. I told him to fetch a half stick and a rope to tie the mule.

"I guess he figured that if I planned to blow the rope and halter to bits along with the animal, he might as well use worn-out equipment. The rope and halter he produced looked anything but stout. But then I was at fault. If had had any notion that mule had enough spirit left to break loose I would have demanded better. The way we both reckoned, afterward, this was rattlesnake country. A mule in that country has an instinctive knowledge and fear of the sound a rattler makes when he is about to strike; and this one may have mistaken the sputtering of the fuse for such a warning. When he reared back the rope broke and he set out on a dead run, sparks flying, for the open door of the barn, some distance away.

"The owner and I could only watch, helpless, from behind the hedge where we had gone for protection. The mule was still a few lengths from the barn when the charge exploded."

SADDLE GALLS

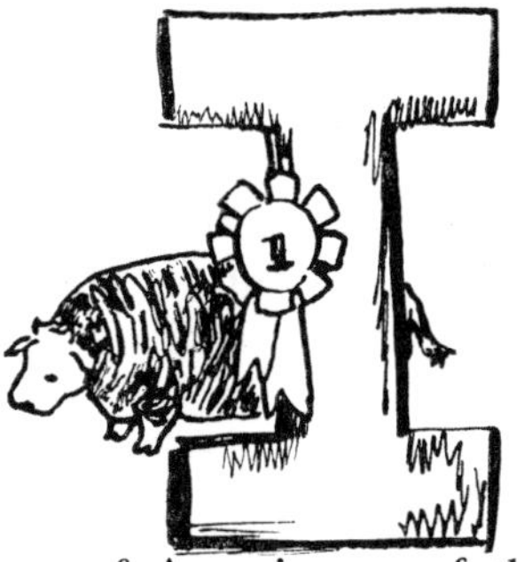

I SUPPOSE that criticism of such well-meant and well-meaning group programs as those carried out by the Future Farmers of America or of the 4-H club might be likened to making derogatory remarks about such cherished American institutions as Little (or big) League baseball or apple pie. But, as a crotchety old has-been, I will step out on a limb long enough to say that it sometimes occurred to me that we did our young people a disservice by the manner in which we not only promoted but magnified the work and the worth of some of these groups.

I am sure that these organizations do fill a need and that they were of value then, and are now, as a substitute for possible mischief and as an absorber of energy. I hasten to say, too, that I am sure many of the programs have improved and that the problem here, as in all other youth work, may lie largely with the fact that the capable and knowledged adult is too often just "too busy" with his own affairs to be a factor in the planning.

During my observation, it seemed to me that the promoters of such programs sometimes used the children to their own ends and that they often tended to give a youngster false notions and bad instruction concerning the breeding and care of livestock.

Looking through the elaborate records some of these young stockmen were obliged to keep on their squat and well-larded animals, we rarely found mention of gain per pound of corn and no estimate at all of the mountain of feed, and of its cost, that had gone into all the pretty, inedible fat that won the purple and blue ribbons. Obviously, the professional stockman is in business for one purpose, to make a profit. Failure to show this to the future farmer or to the 4-H clubber is to give a false impression and a false lesson in economics. Judges of a livestock show who fail to take into account the cost of production are likewise remiss in their judging.

I recall a considerable scandal that resulted from one club calf show when a sensible and perceptive judge, brought in to select the Grand Champion, chose an animal from among the second prize winners in the prior judging, a rangy little Shorthorn, instead of the "apple on legs" that had been named Blue Ribbon calf. When an effort was made to change rules to show the amount of food consumed per pound of weight, a few misguided fathers (of all people!) juggled their sons' records. As a result, blue ribbons went to the biggest liar instead of to the best stock raiser, a miscalculation that taught the youngsters nothing save the justification of any means to an end.

I was called out once (I had better not say where) to look at an ailing calf supposedly being groomed for a show by a young clubber. The father was a bigwig in the program, the boy a bit on the wild side, just the kind who needed a project to keep him occupied.

But I found the father caring for the calf. Inasmuch as one-fourth of the grade points were to be awarded on the animal's performance in the ring, the poor misguided man, wise to an animal's reaction to odors, had hung the boy's jacket over the manger from which the calf took its daily rations. Most of the kids were more honest, and they did keep busy. Preceding a show, they spent countless hours curling hair and polishing hooves. But whereas these chores may keep a lad or lass more or less occupied, silky ringlets and shining hooves do not make an animal a better calf for either breeding or beefsteak. I admit to being an old fogey, but it seems regrettable that too many livestock shows have gone from the hands of genuine breeders into those of men unable to distinguish between bloodline characteristics and so much spit and polish.

From the ranks of these young people come our farmers and ranchers of the future. Their mentors should be the best available. And yet we all too often come across misleading and even erroneous articles in farm and stockmen's magazines written by self-appointed experts (publish or perish, perhaps), articles which, sad to relate, are read by thousands, both young and older, who put complete faith in any printed word under authoritative-sounding authorship.

The discovery of the so-called miracle drugs during my time of practice would certainly rank in importance with experiments in space. But these, too, we came to see could be dangerous in the hands of both the unknowing and the unscrupulous. Owners were influenced by articles and advertisements, and this was understandable. But we were caught squarely in the middle. Many of these drugs proved excellent when properly used and in moderation. No one of them was the cure-all it was purported to be.

We found ourselves pressured by clients who had read of these magic results. Most large and reputable drug companies avoided making use of this ballyhoo and sold only to veterinarians; but some, less ethical, preyed on laymen on the lookout for panaceas. Consequently, high potency products in unlimited quantities fell into the hands of those untrained in both diagnosis and administration and did a lot of harm. Some, of course, harmed only the owner's bank account. But even a useful drug given to man *or* mule without consideration of such factors as age, weight, or activity can serve in the capacity of a poison. Too frequently we found ourselves faced with an effort to dissuade a client who had read these pitches and who thought we simply had not kept up or were depriving him of their benefit for some economic or other reason.

I am moved to confess that some of us who should have known better were also sometimes caught up in the fanfare. Through the years all sorts of remedies have been offered as cures for sterility in both men and animals. When a "guaranteed" product designed to induce ewes to breed twice a year came out, we grabbed the bait, which probably hit every agricultural town in the United States. We knew one owner who treated all two hundred females in his flock.

As a rule, Mother Nature is the wiser judge, a fact we are sometimes inclined to forget. The ewes came in heat all right, as the gimmick literature promised. But not one of them underwent a second lambing.

Late that fall I was approached by a local druggist. "Hey, Doc," he said, "I've got some stuff here I'll sell you at a bargain. It's guaranteed to double lamb harvest."

"Thanks, but no, thanks," I told him sheepishly. "I've got a lot of the same stuff *I'd* like to sell to *you*."

During my time of busiest practice, the addition of drugs to feed was a comparatively new custom. The practice had certain merits for a single animal; but as herd treatment, it seemed to me, you might as well throw your money on a manure heap and save the expense and trouble of buying and feeding. Claims to the contrary, few drugs serve as a preventive, and sick animals, that need the drugs, may well be too sick to eat the rations.

Some of these touted drug additives I found to be genuinely frightening. Most were labeled according to regulation with printed warnings. But I have yet to find many feeders who bother to read the fine print on any sack or package. And who is to check on the middleman or consumer to see that the flesh of an animal or fowl is not consumed within the twenty-four to forty-eight hours specified? The steer fed stilbestrol (diethylstilbestrol) for breakfast in his corn chop may well be tonight's filet. I am obliged to admit there may be a few drawbacks to the system we think of as completely free enterprise.

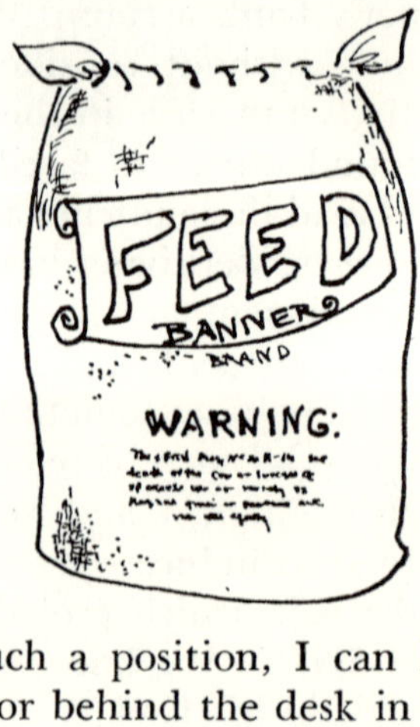

Never having been in such a position, I can hardly know how it is with the administrator behind the desk in Washington, D.C., who must move men about the country like pawns in a chess game. But it did seem sometimes that the U.S. Department of Agriculture wasted a good deal of trained manpower by just plain red tape. The "work measurement program" would stand as a prime example. I do not know how it is done now, but the measurement requirement came to seem not only a waste of time and energy better spent but an invitation to the unscrupulous (or exasperated) field man as well.

I think the program must have been initiated in the early Sixties. At least that was the time of my introduction to it. I suppose that someone, somewhere, may have theorized that we would goof off less if we were obliged to account for the number of units of time consumed by each and every function. In Nevada, where we frequently drove for a half day in order to perform a fifteen-minute job, this obligation appeared especially foolish. One of our more important functions as testers, too, was to sell whatever government program we were working on. For this reason, we found it a good practice to drop in at remote filling stations or stores, have a cup of coffee with whichever ranchers happened to be loafing there, and shoot the breeze about their livestock.

We knew local administrators who were sent back East at taxpayers' expense solely to learn how to fill out these forms so that they could come back to teach other people to teach us. In theory, we worked an eight-hour day. If the sum of the time accounted for fell short of eight hours, we found the returned forms red-penciled as though we were fourth-grade kids. Those who cared enough to make hours and jobs balance could only juggle the figures, and I did not much blame them. I was an old codger by then; I knew I was doing an adequate and honest job and I thought I knew best how to do that job. Faced with long drives, I started early. After driving and working all day, I came home tired out. Then, I wanted to sit down and read the paper, not fill out reports as to how I had spent each and every quarter hour of my time.

There must have been other field men who were as pokey as I about getting out reports, and about as vague. For, finally, they gave us Fridays off "if needed" to fill out forms. We often tested for tuberculosis at the same time we tested for brucellosis. According to the work management sheet we were to record each change of function, so that someone in Washington (who couldn't care less, probably) would know precisely how many minutes we had spent on each job. Once, just for the heck of it, I faithfully recorded each move.

I had gone out to test six cows, in a home-made stanchion with holding room for only one cow at a time. We secured the cow, I took a blood sample for a brucellosis test, returned to the car with said sample, picked up the tuberculosis syringe, walked back, injected the animal, and put on an ear tag, put number one cow back into her quarters, and brought in number two cow for a repeat performance. My report was timed and accurate, but it looked damned silly. For six cows, I had gone through a total of sixty-three changes of function.

On another occasion, one of the helpers on a job was injured by a chute bar and I had to stop work in order to render first aid. In order to account for my time with some degree of accuracy, I made a note of this. Obviously the report was read; for I was officially accused of being "sarcastic." We went along with the reports because we were obliged to do so; but they must have looked pretty sorry sometimes if they were analyzed in terms of accomplishment. One of my colleagues, for example, might be called out to inspect a flock of ten thousand sheep, known as "units," whereas *I* might well have spent the same amount of time on only ten head of cattle. After a while, you developed a tendency to simply set down the first figure that popped into your head. To paraphrase Field Marshal Montgomery: had the program lasted much longer, the department would have run out of paper.

Although I do not question the fact that they do a very great deal of good, one organization that sometimes works against the veterinary as well as the human medical profession in its necessary research is the Society for the Prevention of Cruelty to Animals. I have never known a practicing veterinarian to be cruel to an animal. If he did not like animals, it goes without saying, he would hardly be in the business of administering to them. Few people are aware that the American Veterinary Medical Association has strict guidelines concerning any abuse of animals used and purchased for laboratory work, as well as theft of animals for the purpose of sale to research laboratories. Biologists who buy animals must know the source.

I suppose that any veterinarian, as well as medical doctor, is occasionally handicapped and frustrated by quackery in the profession. I have mentioned some of these people in earlier chapters. As does the human medical quack, the DVM counterpart lives off the difficult and the incurable. We found, often, that it was better to treat the seemingly incurable in some manner, in order to circumvent if possible the "sure cure" that might stand in the way of nature's possible miracle. Not infrequently we were asked, "Why don't you take *after* those fellows?"

We knew a Nebraska veterinarian who tried. The pseudo-doctor was found guilty, and fined twenty-five dollars, which fine he cheerfully paid, and then went back to vaccinating hogs with his useless, cut-rate medication. We also knew a druggist in Woodward, Oklahoma, who wrote the state veterinarian in an effort to stop a shyster from selling an entirely valueless blackleg vaccine. He received the following reply, "Well, we just might be able to get him if some time he fails to pay sales tax on the stuff."

I would like to air one policy complaint: I have never been able to quite understand the custom of allowing practicing veterinarians to decide who should or should not be admitted into a particular state in order to practice veterinary medicine. I have known more than one capable graduate to fail a state examination again and again in his effort to obtain a license to practice in some state of his choice. Is it not unjust to flunk an applicant for other than professional knowledge reasons?

I do not know how it is now. I know that at least one state, some years ago, maintained a policy of licensing each year only

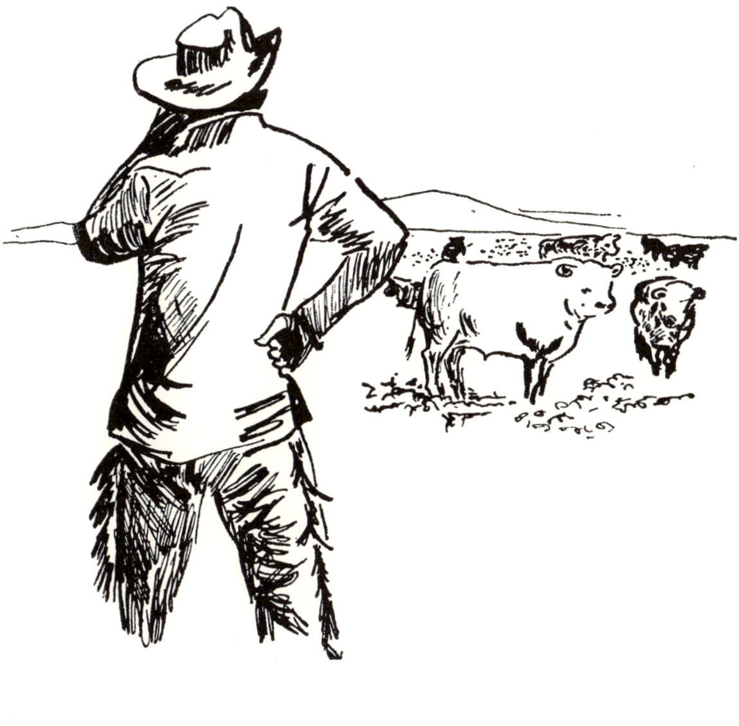

as many veterinarians as the state association had lost that given year or the year previous. Some states, on the other hand, accepted the national board examination results and waived the state examination altogether. This semed to make sense. I realize that such governing laws were passed in order to protect the livestock industry by keeping out the unqualified, and of course this was right. But in some instances I think the veterinarians themselves acted as a kind of union to keep out competition.

As does the debater who takes advantage of his position in the chair to air all of his grievances before he yields his place to another, I would like to say in closing that I think we make a mistake when we upset the ecology of a region by such acts as the killing and poisoning of coyotes, eagles, mountain lions, and various predators. Without such balance, designed by nature, deer and rodents may well multiply to pest proportions. Kill off all the rattlesnakes, as W. C. Fields might have remarked, and you are left with too many children.

AS USEFUL AS TITS ON A BOAR

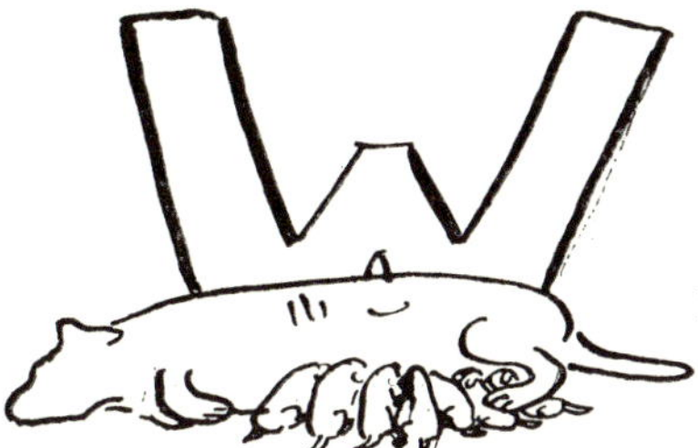

WERE I TO BE GIVEN another start in veterinary medicine, I sometimes think I would make a specialty of genetics. It has occurred to me that a veterinarian could all but make a living off the idiosyncrasies (or errors) of animal breeders influenced by the economic desires and/or whimsies of public demand. Some of these are pretty sad.

One example, understandable enough I suppose, has to do with the breeding of super milk-producing cows, mentioned in an earlier chapter. Too often the end result is milk fever, or bovine mastitis, an inflammation of the udder. Faced with this ailment during practice, I had occasion to remember a young professor in the School of Agriculture in the late Twenties in Manhattan, Kansas, who maintained that we could learn a thing or two about genetics by following the high-producing cow into the slaughterhouse, where she wound up all too soon. The heart and liver, he noted, were simply not big enough to bear all that burden of production.

Whereas I am no trained geneticist, it seems to me that some selectivity in breeding is based on little more than fad and fashion. For all that we as doctors were beneficiaries of some of this foolishness, it seemed in some cases unreasonable and pointless, if not downright inhumane. According to standards set up by someone who, surely, bore little love for dogs, the nose of a purebred bulldog must have a "tip set back deeply between the eyes." As a result, the nose of the hapless animal has been pushed up so far through years of selectivity that it almost literally catches rain. The more apt a bulldog to win best-of-show, the more subject is he to sinus disturbances. Nor can I see that the mashed-looking nose does much to add to his general pulchritude. An uglier face would be difficult to conjure. One wonders why. Perhaps a bull pup was born back along the line somewhere, someone thought the pup was cute, and so the characteristic was passed along as an essential.

Incidentally, the words "purebred" and "thoroughbred" are often confused and misused. Whereas the former may be applied to many species of animals, the word "thoroughbred" is generally applicable solely to horses. Indeed, the word "Thoroughbred," with a capital T, identifies one of a breed of race horses, developed in England by crossing European mares with Arabian stallions.

An instance even more cruel than that of the bulldog is that of the Boston Terrier. In adherence to the puzzling rule that the ideal Boston must be equipped with wide shoulders and narrow hips, breeders have concentrated on these features to such an extreme that few purebred toy Boston bitches are able to bring about a natural delivery.

Nor is horse breeding immune from selective peculiarities. Down the years, we have come to judge a racing colt (and also to price him) on the basis of how fast his sire could run. The will and the ability to run are all-important, with too little thought given, it seems to me, to the fact that said sire and perhaps his sire before him may have run faster than he was physically constructed to run.

Has he the stamina, the heart, the lungs, the legs to stand the strain? Or must he retire all too soon to pasture? As do the heavy-producing cow, and, all too often, the hard-hitting, go-getting business man, he may break down under the demands society has placed upon him. A race horse may reach the top by winning a few of the right races, retire, and command a tremendous stud fee because of his successes. But is he, really, a better animal for this fact?

Personally, I would make a poor out at parimutuel betting. I have seen many races where I would have placed my money on the handsome, sturdy horse that showed good behavior and good characteristics of build. I would have lost almost every time to the backers of the high-spirited, nervous stepper.

According to the rules for standards, the Clydesdale horse, a Scottish breed of strong, sturdy draft animal, must have a feathering of hairs along the backs of his legs. I would like for someone to tell me how these decorations benefit. Outside a cocklebur or sticktight country, I suppose the feathers do him no harm. But neither so far as I can see do they add anything to either his appearance or his value.

I have observed over the years that the popularity of most breeds of animals runs to fads, as do dress and hair styles of the human race. Even varieties of chickens wax and wane in fashion. In the Midwest, a quarter of a century or more ago, for example, the Rhode Island Red hen was prized for her beautiful plumage, removed in any case before she went into the cooking pot or skillet. Later, the New Hampshire Red relegated her to second place. We saw fads in horses, cattle, dogs, sheep, and even hogs and cats prevail for a time and then give way to other fancies.

One fad I found puzzling was that for the Palomino saddle horse. By the end of World War II, the Palomino was in his heyday. With his long flaxen mane and tail, the animal was, indeed, a showy creature. I recall a farmer in Illinois who owned a Palomino stallion, of which he was very proud.

"He's a beauty," I agreed. "But what is he, really? Was he bred for work, or for saddle?"

The owner of the animal bristled with ill-concealed indignation. "He was bred for his mane and tail," he informed me coldly. "Where have you seen such color?"

"Well, if it's color you want," I was inclined to say, "why not black, or blue, with purple or pink or green appendages?"

It occurred to me then and it still seems to me that the Palomino, so-called, embraced characteristics of *both* work and saddle, and that this particular fellow for all his beauty of appearance showed more of the former traits than of the latter. Nor was there ever, so far as I know, complete accord among breeding associations as to Palomino color. One might, for instance, insist upon pink skin, whereas another would not tolerate so much as a suggestion of pink in the shading.

Another widespread example of notional selectivity, it has occurred to me, lies with Hereford or white-faced cattle. This breed appears to do all right in such climates as the cool and frequently cloudy English countryside from which it came. But I have often thought we made a mistake when we spread them out over Western ranges blessed by an abundance of sunshine. Testing for brucellosis in Nevada, we rarely brought as many as two hundred head of Herefords together without finding several cases of that nasty ailment we called cancer eye. We occasionally operated, but frequently too late to stop the spread of the disease. That the condition is brought about, or encouraged, by the reflection of the sun's rays on the white face has long appeared self-evident. And yet we continue to stock sunny Southwest ranges with purebred Herefords. Selective breeders of Hereford cattle could have retained all of their many desirable characteristics with other than a white face.

A red face, or even a roan, would seem more sensible. Of what use to a cow, or to her owner, is a white face that may spell the animal's doom or send her prematurely to the slaughter house, where she may well go into the tank as fertilizer? An alarming number of the animals, we were to discover, found their way into processing plants that dealt with local trade and had no meat inspection whatsoever. This seems poor economy as well as dangerous business.

I was around sixteen years of age, as I recall, when I had my first introduction to Hereford cattle. Because the major portion of Dad's half section of land in southeast Kansas was pasture and meadow land, cattle made up the greater share of the livestock. At first all of our cattle were Shorthorns. One reason for this was that our neighbors had Herefords, and the two breeds were easier to distinguish at a distance. But the other, and principal reason was that despite the fact that Dad had grown up in Herefordshire, England, where Herefords originated, he preferred Shorthorn build. (Shorthorns came from Durham.) He always referred to Herefords as "droop-rumped."

A Shorthorn can be red, roan, or white, and we had all three. We changed bulls about every two years and bought as good as we could afford. One year, I remember, we bought a roan bull, but we had a good deal of trouble with him. For some reason, a roan is a chronic fence crawler, and this one and all of his offspring had a tendency to be "breachy." Maybe this fact had something to do with Dad's switch to Herefords; but I believe it was mainly to get away from so much calving trouble. A Hereford calf is smaller than most breeds at parturition.

One unforgettable time, we lost seven head of cattle at one time to blackleg, a terrible setback. A soilborne disease, blackleg generally attacks animals between the ages of six and eighteen months. These cattle had been running on alfalfa, and I suppose the bacteria must have somehow got into the soil there. Although little was known then (at least by us) concerning the source and nature of the disease, Dad had the sense to move the stock. Even so, we lost six calves and the current bull in a forty-eight hour period.

Our neighbor, Jake Elliott, who claimed to have observed a kind of inoculation during a sojourn in western Kansas, did some "vaccinating" for us. He made an incision in the back of each animal's leg and inserted a cotton swab, as I recall, saturated with some dark-colored medication that resembled iodine. Although blackleg spores are known to live for years in the soil, we escaped further loss. Whatever the reason, we attributed this miracle to Jake's skill and knowledge.

Jersey blood entered our herd by way of a black cow named Bessie, purchased from a local M.D., and her descendants down the years ranged in color and through various patterns and combinations of black and roan to the shade of pale tea. Bessie was a prolific producer of both calves and milk and a great pet, as were some of her daughters. But in some of these offspring, I am bound to say, the watered-down, Shorthorn-Jersey coalition produced a milk of so delicate a blue that we were wont to say you could drop a dime to the bottom of the pail and see whether heads or tails had come uppermost.

During practice, I came to be amused by the strong feeling of aversion the Jersey breed engendered among raisers of beef stock. Ranchers in the vicinity of dairies that might have a Jersey bull kept a sharp lookout lest he come calling on their Herefords. "I don't know why anyone would even milk a Jersey," an Oklahoma rancher remarked to me once, "unless he was too proud to milk a goat."

Even after we changed to Herefords, a few heifers had to be helped each spring with calving. A calf had to be turned, a uterus was thrown, or a vagina gave trouble. I remember especially a rankly amateurish performance when I was in the eighth grade, my first awkward solo experience with animal obstetrics.

While in the process of delivering her second calf, the heifer suffered an inverted and prolapsed uterus. We had, of course, no anesthesia to prevent her straining against any and all efforts to replace the organ. It has always seemed to me that the most taxing physical labor a veterinarian performs is playing midwife to horses and cattle. Both species will fight you to a standstill in instinctive rejection.

"She'll never make it," Dad said. "She'll be dead by morning."

"Could I try?" I ventured.

He shrugged. "Go ahead," he said. "You can't do any harm, I reckon."

Having washed the organ in a creosote dip so strong it's a great wonder it didn't dissolve in the bucket, I pushed it back into place. I have wondered if perhaps the strong creosote acted as a kind of local anesthetic. In any case, the organ remained. The heifer not only lived, she delivered other calves naturally. I still do not know why she lived. Perhaps she had simply not reached the end of her allotted span.

"Never wash a prolapsed uterus," a college professor advised, years later. "Just pick off the hay and surface dirt and shove the organ into place if you can." A secretion on the surface, he maintained, contained a natural antiseptic against bacterial infection.

I offer one tip to those practitioners who have not stumbled onto the improvisation for themselves: There is nothing that beats an aluminum scoop, a common farm tool in corn country, for picking up a thrown uterus, a heavy organ. Such a tool is light, easily cleaned, and rust-proof. A farm, as I have said, is not a hospital. Sometimes you have to make use of that which is at hand. For instance, in cases of extreme emergency, baling wire ("Mormon buckskin") can be used as a suture for a prolapsed uterus or vagina. And strong coffee, it goes without saying, is a fair stimulant for either human or animal.

While we are on the mundane subject of thrown uteri, I would like to say that hogs and chickens should be kept well away from the straining animal lest the organ be damaged or eaten. In Nebraska, where winters were cold, we learned to advise farmers against allowing the organ to freeze before we could reach the scene. A thrown uterus is not a pretty sight, but it is a common one, we used to tell the students with whom we came in contact; and veterinary medicine, as well as its human counterpart, is nothing for the squeamish.

No more than a quarter of a century ago, most hog farmers raised a specific breed of hog, such as Duroc Jersey, Poland China,

Hampshire, and so forth. In grade school agriculture classes, we were taught to distinguish between breeds according to build and color. Then, and later, show hogs at the county fair, where we were lectured by our instructors on field trips, were great, grunting blobs of fat. The more avoirdupois a sow carried about on her abbreviated shanks, the more likely was she to take home a purple ribbon.

But then the scene changed. Housewives began to demand lean bacon; slim hams (called cat hams) replaced heavy loins and shoulders. Lard gave way to vegetable fats, and then to oils. Purebred hogs became a hardly known quantity. When we were in practice in Nebraska corn country, a certain forward-looking genetics outfit in Illinois devised a successful scheme for keeping background records of herds, in order to supply each individual raiser with the best possible boar each year for his particular herd. Some of these boars were odd-looking fellows, nothing a show judge would hang a ribbon on. But this was "planned parenthood," and it worked remarkably well.

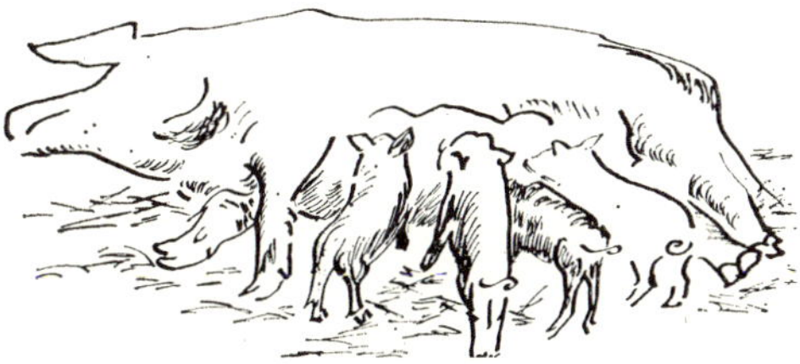

And now I may as well explain the title of this chapter. The oft-repeated phrase "as useless as tits on a boar" may be descriptive enough in characterizing a good-for-nothing, but it lacks an element of truth. In reality, the number of rudimentary tits on the belly of a boar pig is accepted in the trade as an indication of the size of the litter he may be expected to sire, such equipment being considered a trait likely to be passed on to his progeny. The more tits his female offspring show the more apt they are to produce large litters. Twelve to fourteen are looked upon as a good average, and some sows sired by a generously endowed boar may show as many as twenty. Entire breeds have fallen by the wayside because of too-small litters.

A good endowment may be useful to the boar as well. Blessed with a fair number of such extrusions, he may escape castration and so avoid the misfortune of putting in an appearance prematurely on the breakfast table.

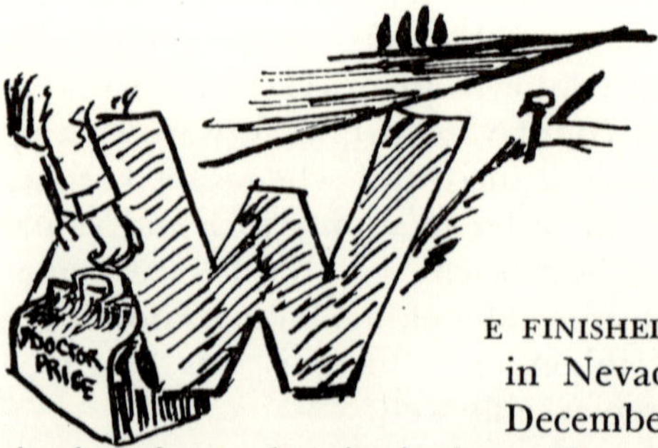

E FINISHED our work with brucellosis in Nevada in the fall of 1965. In December of that year I received a citation from the Agriculture Research Service of the Animal Health Division of the United States Department of Agriculture for "superior performance as district veterinarian in Nevada in work toward the eradication of brucellosis." I say this in all modesty. As I have stated previously, no disease, either animal or human, can be said to be eradicated. It can only be brought under some kind of control. And this was by no means a single-handed accomplishment. As I have already said, my wife Hazel and some others were of inestimable help, and we enjoyed excellent cooperation from all concerned in the project.

A move was forthcoming. Again I was faced with retirement. This time I had reached the stage in life where I wanted only part-time work, a commodity unavailable in the Bureau of Animal Health. The inspection branch of the Poultry Division of Consumer and Marketing Service, I knew, made use of older veterinarians on a part-time basis, as substitutes in poultry processing plants. The work, I thought then, would be seasonal, winter work.

Having worked with poultry in the field both as practicing veterinarian and for the Disease Eradication Division in the Thirties, I felt somewhat familiar with the various ailments a chicken is heir to. Also, I was curious as to how much progress had been made in poultry disease control in thirty-odd years. We had talked of a move to Anderson Island in Puget Sound in Washington State. The west coast area boasted several such plants. It occurred to me that this would be a good base of operation. And so in November of 1965 I went to Turlock, California, for a period of poultry inspection training in an Armour and Company Plant.

My training came to an abrupt and near-disastrous climax. A few days before I was to have returned to Nevada to make the move to Anderson Island, I slipped on a bit of chicken fat on the processing room floor, fell, and suffered a fractured vertebra.

Following my recovery, we moved to Washington. My assignments began that summer, with orders coming out of the San Francisco office. Sometimes, because of a death or illness in a regular inspector's family, I was obliged to go on short notice. One early assignment came on a weekend, with no explanation. The plant was in Idaho. The regular inspector was no longer available for the job, I was told, and a permanent replacement would not arrive for a week. Could I take over meanwhile?

The plant would be open and in business early on Monday morning. There was no time to drive. I donned my metal back brace and flew. On Sunday night I checked in at a motel near the plant. The proprietor who showed me to my room, inquired as to the nature of my business.

"I'm a veterinarian," I told her. "I've come to substitute as an inspector for a week or two at the poultry processing plant."

She gave me a long look. "What an odd coincidence, Doctor. The other inspector lived here, too. He committed suicide on Friday."

For a variety of reasons, my career as a poultry inspector did not last long; but it did result in a few benefits. I came to have a healthy respect for the industry and for its employees. Poultry processing is hard, confining work, assembly-line style, and it begins early in the morning. Live poultry moves at night. Generally we found the trucks waiting at five o'clock or so, when the plants opened.

Only in extreme circumstances can the line be shut down. Nor, save for routine, timed breaks, can an employee leave the progression. Workers draw good pay and they earn every penny. The best plants, I found, were those in which employees (largely women) had become career people. While not classed as skilled laborers, these were in fact highly skilled. Many of the women in the older, established plants were housewives who had worked as trimmers, cutters, drawers for eight to ten years. Several had put children through school with their earnings. I could not help wondering whether these young people realized the day to day pressure to which their mothers were subjected. In any one plant, I found a few employees who could do several or all jobs on the line and do them commendably.

As with most people who work together as a team, the employees knew a good deal about each others' private lives. Obliged to throw a team together one day to kill some fifteen thousand birds, the foreman of one plant discovered to his dismay that the new man in the killing room, armed with a sharp knife, had been stationed side by side with an employee who was keeping company with the new man's wife. Actually, the processing of fifteen thousand chickens is not considered a big day's work. Some of our largest days consisted of as many as thirty-one or thirty-two thousand birds. Rules were strict and rigidly adhered to. Plants were kept immaculately clean.

One fact continues to puzzle me. As a veterinarian, I was naturally interested in the indications in the birds I rejected. But I was amazed to find that there was no way at all to trace the disease back to the source from which the poultry had come, no correlation of field work with processing plant inspection. Under the old B.A.I. we had a free exchange of information between workers in the field and the men in packing plants and this seemed right and as it should be. Inspecting veterinarians were transferred back and forth between plant and field in an effort to trace the diseases back to the farm where the animals had originated. It occurs to me that we erred when we separated the divisions of animal health and of meat inspection. Surely the two should work together for the highest benefit to the consumer.

It just didn't seem to make sense that traceback from processing plant to ranch or farm was all but non-existent. Indeed there seemed in some cases a deliberate conspiracy to keep the source a secret. "No, we don't know whose chickens we're killing," I was told in no uncertain terms. "If *you* knew these birds came from Bill Jones's flock and Bill got a reputation for sending in unhealthy birds, this might ruin him. And it might also influence your judgment."

This kind of theorizing seemed poor business. There we

were, in a position to point out to Bill Jones that his chickens were showing a high incidence of *leukosis* or of air sac infection, so that he could get busy with his veterinarian and clean up the ailment. And yet we weren't even allowed to know where the disease came from.

This was all good experience, but there were other drawbacks. The work was seasonal as I had expected. But it was largely summer seasonal. I was called upon to substitute for vacationing veterinarians who wanted their holidays, naturally enough, during good weather. To be sure I had weekends off. But a portion of those days were frequently spent on the roads, going to or coming from some town where the plant was located. Because of the unconventional working hours, I often traveled by camper, preparing my own meals, or I ate in overnight diners.

On the first day of May, 1968, I retired for the third time. But I was still restless. I felt transplanted geographically, a fish out of water. Northwest summers, as I had anticipated, were pleasant enough. I could cut wood and make garden. But when the rains came, time hung heavy on my hands. I yearned for open, agricultural country, for the sight and sound of livestock, for a people who spoke my language. In April, 1969, I returned to Nebraska, to my old stomping grounds. Presently I went back to work, part-time, for Wisner Veterinary Clinic, a clinic manned by Dr. William Schaulis, Kansas State, 1958, and Dr. Del Heftie, Iowa State, 1963, with Denny Gentrup, a local boy, as helper; and a rare combination of bookkeeper, office manager, purchasing agent, telephone operator, radio operator, medicine mixer, syringe repairman, janitor, and chief dispatcher by the name of Ed Richards. Denny and I thought up some other names for Ed when he was having trouble getting all the calls fitted into a day and dispatched us out over the noon hour to rope, tie, and castrate seventeen five-hundred-pound bulls.

All four of the above are fine individuals, dedicated to serving the public. Some day in the distant future when they, too, are nearing the end of the trail they can sit down and without apology to the world say truthfully, "We did the best we could."

Now that I have the leisure to look back, my working years seem to have passed with inconceivable rapidity. Even the worst years were not without multiple compensations. The bad times, the early deprivations, were far more taxing for Hazel than they were for me. She worked as hard as I did, and handled public relations with clients as I never could have done. It was she who held the family together. She took calls and got them straight, kept the records, accommodated such animals as were brought in, calmed hysterical pet owners, sterilized instruments, mixed and dispensed drugs, lent a hand when needed in the administration. Withall, she retained her sense of humor. We still laugh together over the funny things that happened.

Earlier, as a matter of economics, most veterinarians' offices were at home, as was ours. This not only saved renting office space, it eliminated the necessity of hiring a girl to take calls, an expense we could not have afforded for a long time. If a beginning, single veterinarian were to ask my advice, I would say first off, "Marry a woman who does not insist upon meals on time nor mind night calls, one who is willing to launder work clothing saturated with barnyard and operating filth, who does not object to the smells you bring home, the unfragrant odors that permeate the house she lives in, the car she rides in, the skin of the man she calls husband." A car dealer once told me that he had to deodorize and disinfect any car I traded in, before he could show it to prospects.

Veterinary practice is a seven-day-a-week enterprise, for both the doctor and his wife. We knew a very few vets who knocked off when the fish were biting. We always felt we owed it to our clients to stay on the job. When a solicitor for some sort of labor survey stopped by the house, once, and asked how many hours of work a week we averaged, Hazel told him truthfully, "About eighty." He thought she was pulling his leg.

In the half century since my graduation from high school, we have seen the entire economic picture in this country undergo a metamorphosis. I frequently remember a prognostication made by one of my high school teachers, the late T. B. Henry, concerning our future. "You boys will see more social changes in the next half century," he declared, "than have taken place in total since the beginning of recorded history." The possibility of dying in debt is no longer a dreaded nightmare. For the generation following ours, with credit not only freely come by but urged and promoted, the possibility would appear to be a probability. We look forward to Medicare, to unemployment compensation, to social security, to shorter work weeks and work days, to more leisure than many of us know how to use or to employ.

In a moment of whimsy or of expanded good feeling, I think of how it would be if animals, too, might anticipate some kind of Utopia. Old dogs might go automatically on the program at, say, fifteen, even feral strays. Horses would reach their golden years at age twenty. The cow that had passed her prime, the bull that had outlived his usefulness need not look forward to being canned or corned, nor the worn-out horse to the glue vat. We could all amble happily through the pasture gate together.

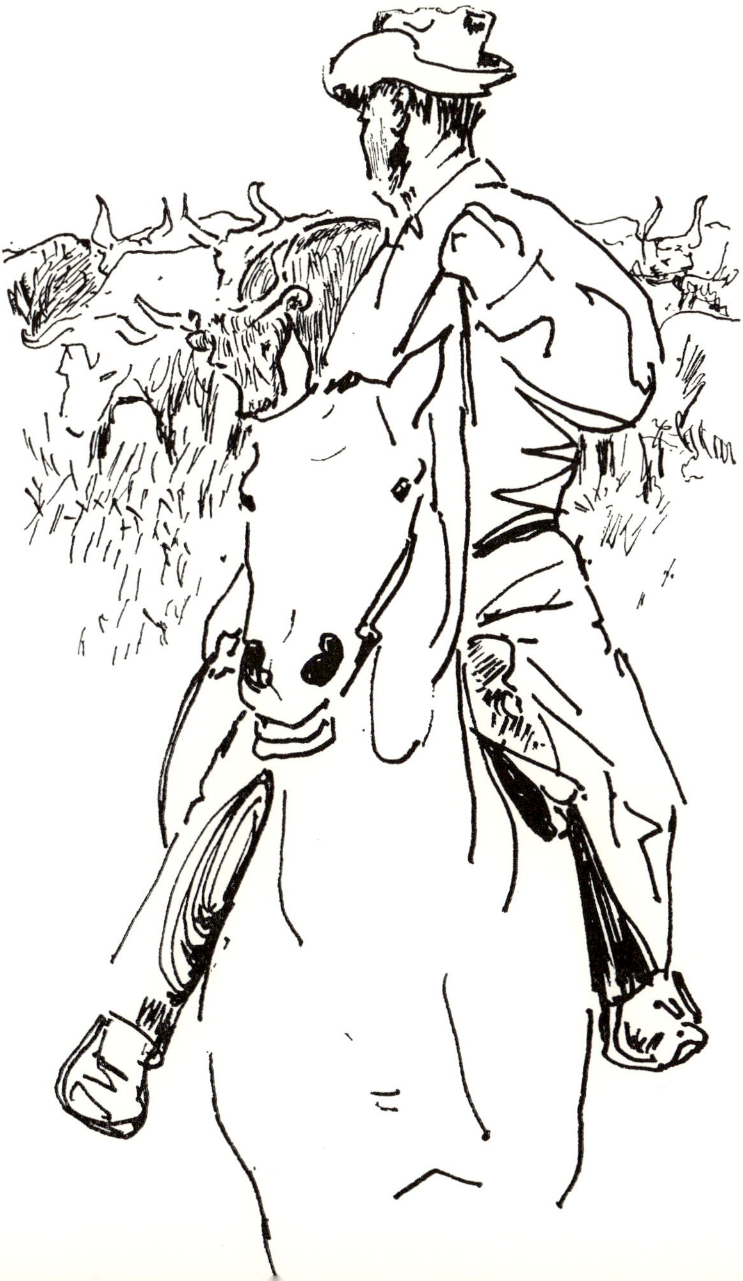